DIALYSIS CHAMPIONS OF THE NEW-ERA THRU THE

KNOWLEDGE POWER

OF "EVIDENCE-BASED PRACTICE RESEARCH"

(Second Edition)

ROSEMARIE ZULETA MSN, BSN, CNN

Dialysis Champions of the New-Era
Thru the Knowledge Power of "Evidence-Based Practice Research"

Copyright@ 2025 by Bluebridge Group Placement Corp.

All rights reserved

No portion of this book may be reproduced, stored in a retrieval system, or transmitted in any form by any means-electronic, mechanical, photocopy, recording, or other-except for brief quotations in printed reviews, without prior permission of the author.

Dedication

This project is dedicated to my family, who have supported me throughout my writing journey.

Specifically, I want to thank my mother, who has put up with my long hours away from the family and has taken on more responsibilities. Her support has given me the time and motivation to complete my degree and achieve my goals.

Acknowledgement

I am humbled and glad for the opportunity to offer my sincere gratitude to everyone who helped create and publish my book, *Dialysis Champion of the New Era Through the Knowledge Power of Evidence-Based Practice Research*.

First, I want to thank my family for their constant support and encouragement during this journey. Their compassion and understanding have been a continual motivation for me, allowing me to follow my passion and complete this book.

Secondly, I want to convey my heartfelt gratitude to my mentor, Alice Hellebrand, DNP, MSN, CNN, whose advice and knowledge have been priceless. Her intelligent input, constructive criticism, and steadfast faith in my talents have all played critical roles in the development of this book.

Next, I extend my gratitude to the dialysis medical professionals, researchers, and specialists whose relentless work and revolutionary discoveries have paved the path for advances in patient care. Because of their passion and commitment, I have been able to investigate and comprehend the complexities of dialysis, enabling me to share this information with the rest of the world.

I thank my coworkers and friends for their help, encouragement, and insightful perspectives during the writing process. Their friendship and thoughtful discussions have enriched the substance of this book and turned it into a collaborative effort. Their enthusiasm and engagement with the subject inspire writers like me to strive for excellence. Their ideas and passion are deeply appreciated.

Finally, I thank the editing team and publishing professionals who worked tirelessly to turn my manuscript into a published work. Their attention to detail, expertise, and dedication have all contributed to the success of this project. Their commitment to fostering a culture of knowledge and learning has supported the development of the evidence-based approach presented in this book.

Thank you for being a part of this incredible journey.

Sincerely,

Rosemarie Zuleta, MSN, BSN, CNN
07/17/2023

About the Author

My journey to becoming an author of a dialysis book did not begin overnight. I started my career in nursing at Chinatown Dialysis Center in the US in 2009. Like many Filipino nurses, I arrived in the US as a qualified nurse who needed to explore the Dialysis Nursing Program to be eligible to become an experienced dialysis nurse in the US.

The first half of the year was a rough go for me. It was challenging to adjust to a new position and setting, and it was unpleasant to have to confine my practice to that context. Later, I went to work for a dialysis healthcare company, Dialyze Direct, where I remained until I was offered my current position. Because there are usually other Filipino coworkers in whatever department I have worked in, I have always felt like an integral part of the team.

In my opinion, renal nursing is a dynamic field with plenty of room for growth, improvement, and its share of challenges. Hospitals have several care units, such as those for chronic, acute, and peritoneal patients. Throughout my career in renal nursing, I have taken advantage of many secondment possibilities, working temporarily elsewhere with the approval of my management and the understanding that my original job would be reserved for me upon completion.

In my nursing career, I have rotated between acute dialysis and renal ward nursing, renal vascular access coordination, renal research nursing, and leadership responsibilities in outpatient dialysis. At the facility where I work, there are subspecialist nursing positions for home therapies, renal anemia, quick assessment, outpatient day cases, and conservative management.

I engage with various CKD patients daily and collaborate closely with their primary care physicians and renal consultants. I work with them to organize medication adjustments and requests for further evaluations. This was a brand-new capability for me, and it was also a previously identified weakness. Therefore, I have focused on developing my capacity for clear and compelling expression through writing and other forms of communication.

I asked for input from our consultants on how well I communicated with my primary care colleagues through letters and texts. The uncertainty surrounding advanced nursing practice is another difficult aspect of my job. Given that patients on chronic dialysis are often stable and their clinical issues are very prevalent, this may seem ironic and atypical for a conventional renal outpatient treatment.

Renal dialysis nursing can be demanding and rewarding; therefore, it is critical to identify these issues and act quickly.

One of my most outstanding achievements was authoring and publishing my first book on dialysis. In my book, I wanted to show that there is life to be had, and that it can be good, even while on dialysis. I drew on my extensive medical training and experience in dialysis departments to address common concerns about the treatment, including how it may affect the patient's ability to eat normally, engage in physical activity, and participate in social events.

I described the dialysis process in detail, including the many treatment options available, the benefits and drawbacks of a kidney transplant, and the potential adverse reactions. Since dialysis impacts the whole family, I shared the humor, fortitude, and successes of families who have successfully confronted the obstacles of dialysis, offering genuine insights into how relatives may manage and prosper together.

The result is a motivational, actionable handbook that teaches dialysis patients and their loved ones how to deal with the challenges of dialysis, face life without fear, and make the most of each day.

As we advance into the future, I want to inspire other aspiring nurses to venture into the dialysis field and become reliable advocates for dialysis patients. My main responsibility as a dialysis advocate is to inform newly diagnosed patients of their choices for dialysis therapy, including home hemodialysis and outpatient dialysis, as well as other methods of kidney care.

Because most patients do not have easy access to their legislators in

Congress, I want to ensure that every patient's voice is heard and that all dialysis patients have the tools to take control of their health. I want to be the first point of contact for those coping with renal illness, providing vital information and emotional support.

I want to aid those dealing with renal illness in adjusting to their potentially dialysis-related new normal. Moreover, as an advocate, I want to provide an entry point for dialysis patients to learn about what is occurring in their bodies, how to manage their health, and what treatment options are available if they need to begin dialysis or contemplate a transplant throughout this life-altering journey. Patients with kidney illnesses will greatly benefit from having someone guide them through getting ready for dialysis.

Preface

This book has been written to address the needs of healthcare professionals working in the nephrology department. It aims to assist these professionals in understanding the principles and applications of current technologies and knowledge in the field. The text is written in simple, easy-to-understand language, making it accessible to anyone with an average or higher level of English proficiency. In this regard, prior advanced knowledge is not required.

This book is suitable for all healthcare professionals, as well as undergraduate and postgraduate students undergoing studies, examinations, or training in nephrology. It covers all clinical aspects of information, supervision, training, and other elements relevant to the nephrology department.

The book is intended for all those involved in the treatment, diagnosis, and care of kidney patients. It will be helpful for individuals pursuing a career in this field, including healthcare professionals, doctors, nurses, and other staff associated with nephrology. Those with a background in medicine or a related field will find this resource valuable for studying the broad range of knowledge available.

The book summarizes the unique challenges that healthcare professionals and patients face in managing and treating various forms of kidney disease. It also raises awareness about the multiple complexities in this field, while preparing readers to make informed decisions about ensuring good kidney health.

The treatment of kidney diseases has undergone significant changes over the past decade. New treatment options have emerged, and technological advancements have revolutionized the treatment process. Outdated ideas must be revised, and existing flaws in practice must be identified and addressed. It is important to overcome the common mistakes that many healthcare professionals unknowingly commit, as doing so will lead to improved patient outcomes and benefit society as a whole.

Writing this book was a formidable task, accomplished through the tireless efforts of the author. Her knowledge, experience, skills, and training have all contributed to the creation of a valuable resource. The clarity of the text will make it easier for you to understand and apply the principles discussed throughout the book.

Contents

Dedication iv

Acknowledgement v

About the Author vii

Preface xi

PART I: Foundations of Renal Health and Dialysis 19

   1: The Role of Functional Kidneys in Preventing Failure 20

   2: Introduction to Dialysis: Process, Purpose, and People 56

   3: Uncovering the Root Causes of Dialysis Needs 79

   4: Managing the Essentials of Dialysis Treatment 104

   5: Inflammation and Pain 133

   6: Clotting Problems and DVT in the Circulatory System 151

   7: Dialysate Temperature and Ph Balance 172

   8: Stroke and HTN 193

   9: Lab Values Involved in Dialysis and Assessment Process . 212

   10: Common Cause of Death among the Dialysis Patients 237

   11: Dialyzable Medications 251

   12: Dialysis Patients Battling with Mental Health Issues 263

   13: Delving More into Quality Assessment and Performance

Improvement on ESRD 280

14: Transforming Lives Through Kidney Transplant 289

15: Benefits Of Medicare Coverage for End Stage Renal Disease (ESRD) People 305

16: Healthy Lifestyle 320

17: HOW TO BECOME AN EFFECTIVE NURSE 341

18: Life Stories of An R.N. Treating Dialysis Patient 352

19: NxStage Home Hemodialysis 360

20: The Future Of Your Health Is In Your Hands And Evolving Modern Dialysis Technology Is Around The Corner 370

PART II: Transforming Healthcare 379

   Introduction 380

   Importance of Case Management 380

   Role of Case Managers 381

   Benefits of Case Management 382

   Comprehensive Care Planning in Dialysis 383

      Tailoring Care to Individual Needs 383

      Ensuring Continuity of Care 384

   Empowering Patients for Self-Management 386

    Lifestyle Modification: Promoting Healthier Living 386

    Self-Management Support: Encouraging Independence 387

Improving Treatment Adherence 388

    Medication Management: Ensuring Safe and Effective Use 388

    Treatment Compliance: Encouraging Consistency in Dialysis 388

    Supporting Lifestyle Modifications: Sustaining Long-Term Health 388

Amplifying Patient Voices 389

Driving Excellence in Dialysis Care 390

Fostering Collaboration for Holistic Care: The Interdisciplinary Dialysis Team Approach 391

    Comprehensive Assessment 392

    Multidisciplinary Collaboration 392

    Goal Setting with Patients 393

    Ongoing Evaluation and Adjustment 393

Ensuring Safe and Effective Medication Use 394

    Medication Reconciliation 394

    Supporting Adherence 394

    Collaboration with Providers 395

    Monitoring and Follow-Up 395

Empowering Patients Through Education ... 395
Disease Education ... 396
Supporting Lifestyle Modifications ... 396
Promoting Treatment Adherence ... 396
Teaching Self-Care Skills ... 397
Team Coordination ... 397
Care Coordination Meetings ... 398
Resource Coordination ... 398
Continuity of Care ... 398

Driving Quality Improvement in Dialysis Care ... 399
Performance Monitoring ... 399
Root Cause Analysis ... 399
Best Practice Implementation ... 400
Patient Feedback and Engagement ... 400
Psychosocial Support and Counseling ... 400
Emotional Support ... 401
Social Support ... 401
Coping Strategies ... 401
Referrals to Mental Health Professionals ... 402

Advocating for Patient Rights 402

    Patient Advocacy 402

    Care Coordination.. 403

    Promoting Health Literacy... 403

    Navigating Ethical Dilemmas 404

Fostering Collaboration: The Interdisciplinary Approach to Dialysis Care 404

    Team-Based Care... 405

    Strengthening Communication Channels................................. 405

    Facilitating Care Transitions 406

    Engaging Patients and Caregivers 406

Transforming Healthcare Through Case Management 407

Medication Reconciliation: Building a Safe Foundation 408

Medication Education: Empowering Patients with Knowledge 409

Medication Coordination: Ensuring Access and Continuity .. 410

Medication Adherence: Overcoming Barriers and Building Habits 411

Case Managers as Agents of Transformation in Healthcare ... 412

Performance Monitoring: Tracking Progress for Better Outcomes

.... 413

Root Cause Analysis: Preventing Problems Before They Recur
.... 414

Continuous Quality Improvement: Embedding Excellence in Care 415

Patient Feedback: The Heart of Quality Care 416

Algorithm Overview 417

    Step 1: Assessing Patient Needs 417

    Step 2: Developing Personalized Care Plans 418

    Step 3: Coordinating with Healthcare Providers 418

    Step 4: Monitoring Patient Progress 418

    Step 5: Educating Patients and Caregivers 419

    Step 6: Advocating for Patients' Rights 419

PART I:
Foundations of Renal Health and Dialysis

1:
The Role of Functional Kidneys in Preventing Failure

Let us begin by exploring the kidneys, two remarkable bean-shaped organs nestled in a position known as retroperitoneal, on either side of the spine, just below the ribcage. Each kidney, weighing about 150 grams and roughly the size of a clenched fist, serves as a silent but formidable powerhouse. While their exterior is simple, their internal architecture is a marvel of biological engineering. Within each kidney lies a complex network of over a million microscopic filtering units called nephrons, the true workhorses responsible for their incredible capabilities.

Their most famous role is that of a sophisticated filtration system. Every day, these two small organs process an astounding 180 liters (about 45 gallons) of blood, diligently sifting out metabolic waste products like urea and creatinine to be excreted in urine. Yet, this is just the beginning of their incredible contribution. The kidneys are also masterful chemists and regulators. They meticulously control blood pressure by releasing the hormone *renin*. They balance crucial electrolytes like sodium, potassium, and calcium, which are essential for nerve function and muscle contraction. They stimulate the production of red blood cells by secreting *erythropoietin* (EPO), ensuring our tissues receive the oxygen they need. Furthermore,

The Role of Functional Kidneys in Preventing Failure

they even play a role in bone health by converting vitamin D into its active, usable form.

Therefore, to see the kidneys merely as waste managers is to miss the masterpiece of their design. They are the master conductors of the body's internal orchestra, ensuring every system plays in harmony. From the pressure within our arteries to the strength of our bones and the very composition of our blood, their influence is profound and constant. Understanding this full scope allows us to appreciate them as the essential, tireless guardians of *homeostasis*, the stable internal environment that is the very foundation of our long-term health and vitality.

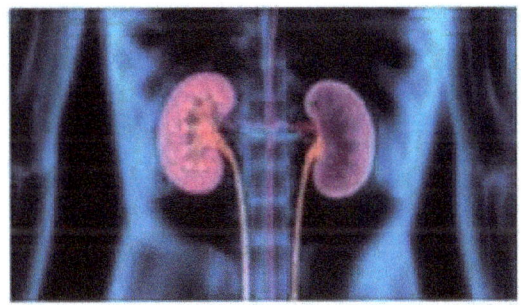

Here are a few essential functions of the kidney:

1. **Maintaining Acid-Base Balance**

    The acids and bases in the human body are always in a delicate equilibrium, as reflected by the pH value. The normal blood pH ranges from 7.35 to 7.45. To keep the body in a healthy range, the kidneys expel excess acids and bases and retain these compounds when the body is deficient. The rate at which your kidneys filter waste is known as the glomerular filtration rate (GFR). This GFR will be lower if your kidneys are injured. Your estimated glomerular filtration rate (eGFR) and various stages of damage are shown by blood testing.[1]

2. **Blood Pressure Maintenance**

Renin is an enzyme produced by the kidneys. Renin transforms angiotensinogen, generated in the liver, into angiotensin I, which is then converted into angiotensin II in the lungs. Angiotensin II constricts blood vessels, causing blood pressure to rise.

When blood pressure is excessively high, the kidneys generate more urine to decrease the volume of liquid circulating in the body and help compensate for the high pressure.

3. **Osmolality Regulation**

The kidneys aid in maintaining the body's water and salt levels. The hypothalamus, which communicates directly

---

[1] https://www.webmd.com/a-to-z-guides/what-to-know-about-stages-chronic-kidney-disease

with the posterior pituitary gland, detects any significant increase in plasma osmolality.

When osmolality rises, the gland secretes antidiuretic hormone (ADH), which stimulates water reabsorption by the kidney and increases urine concentration. These components work together to restore normal plasma osmolality levels.[2]

4. **Vitamin D Activation**

The kidneys produce the hormones calcitriol and erythropoietin. Calcitriol is a form of vitamin D that aids in calcium absorption. The kidneys convert calcifediol into calcitriol, the active form of vitamin D. Calcitriol circulates in the blood and regulates calcium and phosphate balance in the body, which is necessary for proper bone formation. Erythropoietin is a hormone that aids in producing red blood cells. Calcitonin, another hormone secreted by the thyroid gland, works in response to hypocalcemia. This hormone counteracts hypercalcemia and prevents osteoclast activity. It stimulates the deposit of calcium and phosphates into bones.

5. **Removing Toxins and Waste from the Body**

---

[2] https://pubmed.ncbi.nlm.nih.gov/15453232/#:~:text=The%20kidneys%2C%20in%20concert%20with,differ%20within%20each%20nephron%20segment.

The kidneys filter out water-soluble waste products and toxins, excreting them through urine. That is why kidney failure quickly leads to severe intoxication, as waste products accumulate and impair the body's functions.

6. **Measuring Function**

    Various computations and procedures are used to assess renal function. Renal clearance refers to the volume of plasma from which a substance is completely removed per unit of time.

    The filtration fraction is the quantity of plasma filtered through the kidneys. This can be defined using mathematical equations. Because the kidney is a highly complex organ, mathematical modeling has been used to better understand renal function at multiple levels, including fluid uptake and secretion.

The Kidneys: Endocrine Powerhouses for Homeostasis

The kidneys are vital to maintaining the body's internal stability, or *homeostasis*. They act as master regulators for critical processes such as acid-base balance, electrolyte levels, blood pressure, and, crucially, hormone production. When the kidneys fail, this delicate balance is severely disrupted, leading to life-threatening complications. These may include debilitating fatigue, difficulty breathing, widespread swelling (edema), metabolic acidosis, and

The Role of Functional Kidneys in Preventing Failure

irregular heart rhythms (cardiac arrhythmias).

Beyond their renowned filtering function, the kidneys act as sophisticated endocrine organs, producing three essential hormones that are indispensable for homeostasis.

1. Erythropoietin (EPO)

Erythropoietin is the hormone responsible for stimulating the bone marrow to produce red blood cells, which are the primary transporters of oxygen in the blood. The kidneys continuously monitor oxygen levels in the blood passing through them. If they detect low oxygen levels, a condition known as *hypoxia*, they increase the secretion of EPO. This prompts the bone marrow to ramp up red blood cell production, thereby increasing the oxygen-carrying capacity of the blood and restoring normal oxygen levels to the body's tissues. In chronic kidney disease, insufficient EPO production is a primary cause of anemia, leading to the profound fatigue experienced by patients.

2. Renin and the Renin-Angiotensin-Aldosterone System (RAAS)

Renin, which acts as both a hormone and an enzyme, is the crucial first step in a powerful cascade called the **Renin-Angiotensin-Aldosterone System (RAAS)**. This system is the body's primary mechanism for regulating blood pressure and fluid balance. When the kidneys detect a drop in blood pressure or low sodium levels, they release renin into the bloodstream. Renin initiates a chain reaction that results in the formation of **angiotensin II**, a potent molecule with two main effects:

- **Vasoconstriction:** It narrows blood vessels throughout the body, immediately increasing blood pressure.//
- **Aldosterone Stimulation:** It signals the adrenal glands (located on top of the kidneys) to release another hormone, **aldosterone**. Aldosterone then acts on the kidneys, instructing them to retain more sodium and water, which increases blood volume and, consequently, blood pressure over the long term.

3. Calcitriol (Active Vitamin D)

While we often associate Vitamin D with sunlight and diet, it is biologically inert until it is activated, and the final, most critical step of this activation process occurs in the kidneys. The kidneys convert inactive Vitamin D into its active form, **calcitriol**. Calcitriol is essential for maintaining calcium and phosphate balance in the body. It functions by promoting the absorption of calcium from the intestine and regulating its transfer into and out of bone tissue. Without adequate calcitriol, the body cannot effectively absorb calcium, leading to low blood calcium levels and bone diseases like renal osteodystrophy. This hormone is therefore indispensable for maintaining strong bones, as well as proper nerve and muscle function.[3]

How Do Different Foods Good for Kidneys Compare?

The kidneys are small organs in the lower abdomen but play a crucial role in overall health. While some foods support kidney function, others can be harmful. That's why it is important to choose the right foods. A kidney-healthy diet can help kidneys work effectively and protect them from damage.

Blueberries

Blueberries are rich in vitamin C, fiber, and antioxidants. They can help reverse some of the problems caused by chronic kidney disease by reducing inflammation and supporting bone health.

Onions

Onions, like garlic, offer a fantastic salt-free flavoring option, especially when sautéed in olive oil. They contain essential nutrients such as manganese, copper, and vitamins B6 and C. Onions also contain organic sulfur compounds that may reduce the risk of high blood pressure, stroke, and heart disease, as well as quercetin, which helps fight cancer.

Garlic

---

[3]https://www.ncbi.nlm.nih.gov/books/NBK536997/#%3A~%3Atext%3DErythropoietin%20(EPO)%20

Garlic contains an active ingredient that protects kidney health as effectively as some prescription medications. Garlic should be a staple in any renal-friendly diet.

Whole Grains

Whole grains such as oats, barley, whole wheat, brown rice, and quinoa are high in vitamins, minerals, and fiber, promoting digestive and overall health. If you need to limit mineral intake, choose buckwheat or bulgur (cracked wheat), which contain less potassium, sodium, and phosphorus than grains like quinoa and oats.

Red Peppers

Red peppers are rich in vitamin C, a well-known antioxidant. They contain less potassium than many other vegetables, making them suitable for people with kidney disease. They also provide vitamin A, which supports a healthy immune system.

People who wish to keep their kidneys healthy and those with advanced kidney disease must follow a kidney-friendly diet. This is known as a renal diet, which ensures that waste does not accumulate in the blood. This diet is essential for boosting kidney function and preventing further damage.

A Brief Comparison of the Nutritional Foods in a Renal Diet

Experts have recommended restricting the following nutrients in your diet if you are diagnosed with kidney disease.

The Role of Functional Kidneys in Preventing Failure

Sodium

Found in many foods and being an integral part of table salt, this nutrient must be restricted to less than 2,000 mg daily. The problem with damaged kidneys is that they cannot filter out sodium if taken in excess, which then causes the blood levels to rise.

Potassium

Potassium is important for the body as it plays many different roles. However, if there is an underlying kidney issue, its intake must be limited, or it would lead to high blood levels that are dangerous for the body. The recommended limit is less than 2,000 mg per day.

Phosphorus

Found in many foods as a mineral, phosphorus intake needs to be restricted to less than 2,000 mg per day, as a diseased kidney cannot remove excess phosphorus, leading to high levels in the blood.

Protein

This nutrient also needs to be limited if you have kidney disease. The reason is that protein metabolism gives rise to waste products, and damaged kidneys cannot remove this waste effectively.

Following a renal diet does not mean sacrificing flavor or variety. In fact, many delicious and nutrient-rich foods can be enjoyed while supporting kidney health. Some excellent choices include cauliflower, blueberries, sea bass, red grapes, onions, bell peppers, radishes, turnips, egg whites, garlic, cabbage, skinless chicken, buckwheat, olive oil, bulgur, and pineapple. While some nutrients must be monitored closely in a kidney-friendly diet, there is no need to eliminate them entirely. A wide range of low-nutrient alternatives is available, making it easy to maintain a well-balanced and satisfying meal plan.

Adopting a renal diet can be an uplifting experience, filled with delicious possibilities that promote overall health. With mindful choices, individuals can protect their kidney function while enjoying meals that are both nourishing and flavorful.

The Role of the Amount of Water in Keeping Kidneys Healthy

Hydration plays an essential role in keeping your kidneys functioning optimally. While a common recommendation is to drink eight glasses of water daily, actual needs vary significantly from person to person. Factors such as age, physical activity, climate, pregnancy, breastfeeding, and illness all influence the ideal amount of fluid intake.

Water supports the kidneys by helping them flush waste products from the blood through urine. It also ensures proper circulation, enabling nutrients to reach the kidneys efficiently. When the body is dehydrated, kidney function begins to suffer. Even mild dehydration can cause fatigue and impair bodily functions. In more severe cases, it may lead to kidney damage.

It is especially important to stay hydrated in hot climates or during increased physical activity. While the U.S. Dietary Guidelines for 2015–2020 do not set a specific daily water requirement, the United Kingdom's National Health Service recommends six to eight glasses of fluids per day, including those found in food. Keep in mind, though, that this guideline applies to temperate climates. If you live in a warmer region, your body will need more fluids to maintain proper function.

Recommended Amount of Water Intake in Healthy Pediatric, Adult, and Geriatric Populations

Infants

Plain water is not recommended for infants. According to the Centers for Disease Control (CDC), infants may be given additional water in a bottle if the weather is hot, but the primary source of fluids should still be breast milk or formula.

Children after one year

After 12 months of age, children should be educated about the importance of drinking water. They should be encouraged to consume more water daily, especially during warm weather. They should also be taught to prefer water over sweetened drinks and juices.

Adults aged 18 to 30

The recommended daily water intake is 3.7 liters for men and 2.7 liters for women. If a woman is pregnant, an extra 0.3 liters is required. Those who are breastfeeding need an additional 0.7 to 1.1 liters.

Older adults

Older individuals are at increased risk of dehydration. This risk is due to medications, health conditions, loss of muscle mass, and other factors such as reduced kidney function.

There are many advantages to staying hydrated in older adults, such as fewer falls, avoiding constipation, and a reduced risk of bladder cancer in older male adults.

Dehydration in older age contributes to urinary tract infections, kidney failure, and slower wound healing.

Maintaining pH Balance and Hydration in Dialysis Patients

Staying hydrated is essential for everyone, but for individuals with chronic kidney disease (CKD), especially those undergoing dialysis, hydration becomes a delicate balancing act. Healthy kidneys maintain the body's fluid balance by filtering and excreting excess water and waste through urine. However, when kidneys are damaged and lose their filtering capacity, this equilibrium is disrupted, putting patients at risk of fluid overload, a condition

The Role of Functional Kidneys in Preventing Failure

clinically known as hypervolemia.

Fluid overload isn't just about feeling bloated, it can lead to dangerous complications such as high blood pressure, swelling in the legs and arms (edema), difficulty breathing due to fluid in the lungs, and even heart failure. To minimize these risks, dialysis patients are generally advised to limit their daily fluid intake to around 32 ounces (approximately 1 liter). This includes not only water but also ice, soup, fruit, and other fluid-containing foods, which can make the restriction particularly challenging.

Dialysis and Metabolic Management

Dialysis helps replace some of the kidneys' vital functions by removing excess fluid, electrolytes, and waste products from the blood. But dialysis alone is not enough. Individuals on dialysis are also vulnerable to serious metabolic imbalances, particularly in acid-base regulation and electrolyte levels, including potassium, sodium, calcium, and phosphate. Disruptions in these areas can lead to life-threatening conditions, such as cardiac arrhythmias, bone disorders, or metabolic acidosis.

One of the primary goals of managing CKD is to maintain a stable blood pH level, which is crucial for cellular function, enzyme activity, and oxygen delivery. If the blood becomes too acidic or too alkaline, patients may experience fatigue, confusion, muscle weakness, or worse, leading to increased hospitalizations and, in severe cases, death.

The Role of Diet and Dialysis Prescriptions

As CKD progresses, metabolic disturbances become more severe and more difficult to control. This is why treatment must involve a comprehensive and personalized approach. Patients are often guided to follow a renal diet, which typically restricts:

- **Sodium**, to control blood pressure and reduce fluid retention
- **Potassium**, to prevent dangerous heart rhythms
- **Phosphorus**, to protect bones and prevent itchy skin or vascular calcification
- **Protein**, to minimize waste buildup while still supporting muscle health

Each patient's diet is adjusted based on lab results, stage of kidney disease, and whether they are receiving dialysis. Additionally, **dialysis prescriptions**, including session duration, frequency, and dialysate composition, are tailored to each individual's needs. This personalized strategy not only enhances treatment effectiveness but also improves quality of life by minimizing complications like fatigue, cramps, or low blood pressure during dialysis sessions.

Understanding Kidney Disease: A Silent Threat

Chronic kidney disease is a long-term, progressive condition in which the kidneys gradually lose their ability to function. This loss

The Role of Functional Kidneys in Preventing Failure

is often silent in the early stages, with symptoms only becoming apparent after substantial damage has occurred. The disease is typically staged from 1 to 5, with stage 5 (also called end-stage renal disease) requiring dialysis or a kidney transplant.

CKD can affect anyone, but certain populations are disproportionately impacted. Individuals of South Asian, African, and Hispanic descent face a higher risk due to genetic and socioeconomic factors. Additionally, people with diabetes, high blood pressure, obesity, or a family history of kidney disease are more susceptible.

Interestingly, while CKD is common in older adults (65 and above), its progression tends to be more stable and manageable in this group. In contrast, younger patients often experience faster disease progression, potentially due to more aggressive underlying causes or lower adherence to medical care.

Prevention and Early Detection

There is currently no cure for CKD, but early detection and consistent management can dramatically slow its progression. Regular blood and urine tests, such as the glomerular filtration rate (GFR) and urine albumin-to-creatinine ratio (ACR), are critical for detecting kidney damage early. Once diagnosed, patients should adopt lifestyle changes like quitting smoking, exercising regularly, managing blood sugar and blood pressure, and avoiding over-the-counter medications like NSAIDs, which can be harmful to the kidneys.

Healthcare professionals emphasize routine checkups and patient education, which empower individuals to take control of their health and respond to warning signs early. For example, unexplained fatigue, changes in urination, swelling, or persistent itching could signal worsening kidney function.

Acute vs. Chronic Kidney Failure: What's the Difference?

Your kidneys are not only responsible for filtering blood but also play an essential role in regulating blood pressure, producing hormones like erythropoietin (which stimulates red blood cell production), maintaining bone health, and balancing water, salt, and mineral levels in the body.

These vital functions are carried out by millions of microscopic filtering units called nephrons. Each nephron includes a glomerulus, which filters your blood, and a tubule, which processes the filtrate by reabsorbing needed substances and discarding the rest as urine.

When kidney function suddenly declines over a few hours or days, it's referred to as acute kidney failure (or acute kidney injury). Causes may include severe dehydration, infections, trauma, drug toxicity, or reduced blood flow to the kidneys. While frightening, acute kidney failure is often reversible if treated promptly.

The Role of Functional Kidneys in Preventing Failure

In contrast, chronic kidney failure develops slowly and insidiously, typically over months or years. Its causes are more deeply rooted, such as long-term hypertension, poorly controlled diabetes, autoimmune disorders (like lupus), or polycystic kidney disease, and the damage is usually irreversible.

Stages of CKD

An important marker of kidney function is creatinine, a waste product produced when muscles contract. Healthy kidneys remove creatinine from the blood. However, as kidney function declines, blood creatinine levels increase.

The severity of kidney disease is measured by the glomerular filtration rate (GFR), which is calculated using a person's age, gender, and serum creatinine level.

Here are the stages of kidney disease:

Stage 1

Normal or high GFR (greater than 90 mL/min)

Kidneys have mild damage but continue to function normally.

Stage 2

Mild CKD (GFR 60–89 mL/min)

Kidney damage is more significant than in Stage 1, though kidney function remains fairly intact.

Stage 3

Moderate CKD (GFR 30–59 mL/min)

There is mild to severe loss of function, resulting in a decline in the kidneys' ability to remove metabolic waste.

Stage 4

Severe CKD (GFR 15–29 mL/min)

A significant decline in kidney function occurs, and waste removal becomes inefficient.

Stage 5

End-Stage CKD (GFR less than 15 mL/min)

Kidneys are nearing failure or have already failed. Metabolic waste is not being removed, and dialysis is required.

Signs You May Have Kidney Disease

Here are some of the most evident signs that you may be suffering from kidney disease:

Pain in the lower back

When you move or stretch, you may feel localized discomfort near your kidneys that does not go away or worsens. Kidney issues can result in lower back pain, as the kidneys are located on either side of the spine. Back discomfort can also result from infections or kidney obstructions, which may harm the kidneys.

The Role of Functional Kidneys in Preventing Failure

A decreased appetite

You may lose your appetite due to feeling full, being too tired or sick to eat, or because of a buildup of toxins caused by reduced kidney function.

To make urine, healthy kidneys filter blood. Urination problems, such as the desire to pee more frequently or noticing blood in your urine, can happen when the kidneys are not working correctly. Additionally, you may see frothy or bubbly urine, which might indicate that protein is entering your urine due to damaged kidneys.

Fatigue

You may have low energy or extreme fatigue due to a buildup of toxins in the blood caused by impaired kidney function. Anemia, which results from having too few red blood cells, can make you feel exhausted or weak and may also be brought on by chronic kidney disease (CKD).

Itching

If you have dry and itchy skin, you may have a mineral and nutritional imbalance in your blood caused by renal illness. High amounts of phosphorus in the blood may induce itching.

Swelling in hands, legs, or feet

Edema, often known as swelling, can develop in your feet or other lower limbs when your kidneys are not eliminating excess salt and fluid from your body.

Difficulty in breathing

When your kidneys are not draining enough fluid, extra fluid might accumulate in your lungs, making you feel out of breath. Breathlessness may also be brought on by CKD-induced anemia, a deficiency in red blood cells that deliver oxygen.

Abnormal amounts of calcium, phosphorus, or vitamin D

Electrolyte imbalances caused by impaired kidney function, such as low calcium levels or excessive phosphorus, can result in muscle cramps.

Abnormal urine test

Proteinuria, or high protein levels in the urine, is a symptom of renal disease. Protein escapes into your urine when the kidneys are not working correctly. When the kidneys are healthy, protein can re-enter circulation, while waste and fluid are filtered out.

Elevated blood pressure

You may experience elevated blood pressure due to the extra fluid and salt buildup caused by kidney illness. In addition to damaging renal blood vessels, high blood pressure can eventually aggravate

The Role of Functional Kidneys in Preventing Failure

kidney disease.[4]

Can the Current Stage of Kidney Disease Be Established Based on the Presence of Metabolic Wastes Like Creatinine and BUN?

Blood urea nitrogen (BUN) typically ranges between 7 to 20 mg/dL or 2.5 to 7.1 mmol/L. There is no definite value of BUN that alone can diagnose kidney failure. The test is usually done alongside others to support a diagnosis of kidney dysfunction or to monitor how well your medications for kidney disease are working.[5]

Depending on your age, gender, medical history, and other factors, test results may vary. Results may also differ based on the laboratory used and might not necessarily indicate a problem. Always consult your healthcare practitioner to interpret your test results.

An average BUN level considered normal ranges from 7 to 20 milligrams per deciliter (mg/dL). This level can help your doctor assess the health of your kidneys. However, levels higher than 60 mg/dL may be cause for concern.

The ratio of BUN to creatinine in your blood provides a more accurate gauge. BUN to creatinine ratios typically range from 10:1 to 20:1. If the ratio is lower or higher than that, it could indicate

---

[4] https://www.freseniuskidneycare.com/kidney-disease/ckd/symptoms
[5] https://www.freseniuskidneycare.com/kidney-disease/ckd/symptoms

kidney dysfunction or dehydration, respectively.[6]

Various techniques for measuring BUN and creatinine have emerged over time. Most of these are automated and produce clinically accurate and repeatable results.

Urea nitrogen can be measured using one of two techniques. The diacetyl, or Fearon, reaction produces a yellow chromogen with urea, which can be measured through photometry. This method has been adapted for autoanalyzers and typically gives reliable results. However, it has low selectivity, and misleading increases can occur with sulfonylurea drugs or when hemoglobin interferes with whole blood colorimetry.[7]

What Is the BUN Test?

The Blood Urea Nitrogen (BUN) test is a common diagnostic tool used to assess kidney function. It measures the amount of urea nitrogen present in your blood. Urea nitrogen is a waste product that forms when the liver breaks down protein in the body. After its formation, urea enters the bloodstream and is transported to the kidneys, which filter it out and excrete it in the urine.

The BUN test is performed by drawing a small sample of blood,

---

[6] https://www.urmc.rochester.edu/encyclopedia/content?contenttypeid=167&contentid=ur

[7] https://www.ncbi.nlm.nih.gov/books/NBK305/

usually from a vein in your arm. The procedure is quick, typically requiring no special preparation, though your healthcare provider may advise fasting or avoiding certain medications before the test, depending on the broader panel being ordered.

A certain level of urea in the blood is normal. However, elevated levels may indicate that the kidneys are not functioning properly and are failing to excrete waste products efficiently. High BUN levels can be a sign of kidney disease, dehydration, or conditions that affect blood flow to the kidneys, such as congestive heart failure or shock. On the other hand, low BUN levels are less common but can occur in cases of severe liver damage, malnutrition, or overhydration.

What Is the Purpose of a Blood Urea Nitrogen (BUN) Test?

The BUN test is often included as part of a routine health checkup and is typically one component of a **basic metabolic panel (BMP)** or **comprehensive metabolic panel (CMP)**, which evaluate a range of substances in the blood to give a broad picture of your overall health.

Doctors may order a BUN test for a variety of reasons, including:

- **Monitoring kidney function** in patients with chronic kidney disease or those undergoing dialysis.
- **Evaluating acute symptoms** such as confusion, fatigue, nausea, or changes in urine output.

- **Assessing hydration status**, especially in elderly individuals or those with symptoms of dehydration.

- **Checking the effects of medications**, such as diuretics or certain antibiotics, which can affect kidney function.

- **Monitoring patients with heart conditions**, liver disease, or diabetes, all of which can impact kidney health.

- **Guiding treatment decisions** in critical care settings, such as during hospitalization or emergency care.

Changes in BUN levels are typically interpreted alongside other lab values, such as **creatinine**, to provide a more complete assessment of kidney health. The **BUN-to-creatinine ratio** is a particularly useful metric in determining whether kidney impairment is due to pre-renal (e.g., dehydration), renal (intrinsic kidney damage), or post-renal (obstruction) causes.

If you have risk factors for kidney disease, your doctor may order a BUN test as a precaution. Early kidney disease often has no symptoms. However, several factors can increase your risk, including:

- A family history of kidney disease
- Hypertension
- Diabetes
- Cardiovascular disease

The Role of Functional Kidneys in Preventing Failure

If your doctor suspects kidney disease, they may conduct a BUN test based on the following symptoms:

- Frequent urination or insufficient urination
- Fatigue
- Unusual urine appearance (bloody, foamy, or coffee-colored)
- Swelling of the eyes, face, abdomen, arms, legs, or feet
- Vomiting or nausea"[8]

The quantity of urea nitrogen in your blood is determined by a blood urea nitrogen (BUN) test. When your liver breaks down protein, urea nitrogen is produced as a waste product. Your blood carries it, your kidneys filter it out, and your urine excretes it from your body.

Your liver may not properly break down proteins if it is not in good shape. Additionally, unhealthy kidneys may be unable to filter urea effectively. Higher urea nitrogen levels may develop in your body because of either of these issues. BUN plays an essential role in kidney diseases.

Does the treatment during the end stage of renal disease depend on the dialysis machine's parameters like time, volume, and

---

[8] https://my.clevelandclinic.org/health/diagnostics/17684-blood-

BFR to obtain the blood liters processed for the adequacy of the dialysis?

The main factors determining the type of dialysis for people with chronic kidney disease are patient preferences about the treatment that best suits their lifestyle, availability of options within a service, and clinical contraindications.

When we talk about dialysis, two main types of dialysis are available: hemodialysis and peritoneal dialysis.

The factors that patients and caregivers may need to consider about peritoneal dialysis include:

- The ability to carry out dialysis themselves
- The support services they need to carry out dialysis
- Integration of dialysis with work, school, hobbies, and social and family activities
- Opportunities to maintain social contacts
- Possible modifications to their home
- The distance and time traveling to the hospital
- Flexibility of daily treatment, diet, and medication regimens
- Potential changes to body image and physical activities

The Role of Functional Kidneys in Preventing Failure

because of dialysis access points[9]

Adequate dialysis is essential for reducing morbidity and mortality among patients requiring hemodialysis. Kt/V is referred to as the standard marker for dialysis adequacy. Kt/V is modifiable through different factors such as dialyzer type, dialysis frequency, duration of dialysis, dialysate flow rate, and dialyzer blood flow rate (BFR).

BFR is essential for achieving adequate Kt/V in fourth and end-stage chronic kidney failure. Increasing BFR while keeping the same surface area and dialysate flow leads to a 23 percent increase in urea clearance. Hence, lower BFR causes inadequate dialysis outcomes.

If BFR is kept below 250 mL during hemodialysis, it may increase mortality for chronic HD patients. Monitoring the factors that boost BFR is essential, as they help improve the results.

Which is the best nutritional supplement for CKD patients that contains less sugar?

Sugar intake, particularly in the form of fructose, has been linked to renal damage. Fructose metabolism increases uric acid production, oxidative stress, and inflammation, factors that contribute to kidney injury and progression of chronic kidney disease (CKD). Because their compositions are comparable, there is no evidence that sucrose

---

[9] https://pubmed.ncbi.nlm.nih.gov/22536622/

is safer for the kidney than high fructose corn syrup (HFCS). Both forms of sugar may negatively impact renal function over time, especially in individuals with pre-existing kidney impairment.

So far, five epidemiologic studies have directly examined the link between sugar consumption, primarily through sugar-sweetened beverages (SSBs), and CKD. Although most research implies that SSB consumption is associated with an increased risk of CKD, only a few studies have found statistically significant relationships. This discrepancy may be due to limitations in sample size, dietary assessment tools, or variations in population health and lifestyle factors.

Given the potential harm of excess sugar and the need for nutrient-dense options, **CKD patients are advised to choose nutritional supplements with low sugar content, balanced protein, and minimal phosphorus, potassium, and sodium**, especially in later stages of the disease.

Recommended low-sugar nutritional supplements for CKD patients include:

1. **Nepro with Carb Steady® (by Abbott):**

    Designed specifically for dialysis patients, Nepro is low in potassium and phosphorus and includes a controlled carbohydrate blend to minimize blood sugar spikes.

2. **Novasource Renal (by Nestlé Health Science):**

   A high-calorie, low-protein, low-electrolyte formula suitable for patients with fluid restrictions and early-to-late-stage CKD. It contains minimal sugar compared to general nutritional drinks.

3. **Suplena® with Carb Steady® (by Abbott):**

   Formulated for pre-dialysis patients, Suplena is low in protein but offers heart-healthy fats, limited sugar, and reduced levels of electrolytes.

4. **Homemade CKD Smoothies:**

   For a more natural option, smoothies made with unsweetened almond milk, low-potassium fruits (like apples or berries), and CKD-approved protein powders can provide nutrients without added sugars or preservatives.

Important Considerations:

- Always consult a nephrologist or renal dietitian before starting any supplement.
- CKD patients with diabetes should prioritize supplements with low glycemic indexes.
- Supplements should complement, not replace, whole food intake unless medically necessary.

In conclusion, while more research is needed to clarify the exact role of sugar in CKD progression, current evidence suggests minimizing added sugars is beneficial. CKD patients should focus on renal-specific supplements that are low in sugar and tailored to their stage of kidney function and overall health status.

How much water to drink: an integral part of kidney health in pediatric, adulthood, and geriatric stages of healthy people and dialysis patients regarding pH balance and hydration

Be water wise to protect the health of your kidneys. This involves consuming the appropriate volume of water for you. The amount of water you require depends on your age, the environment where you live, how hard you exercise, and whether you are a dialysis patient, adult, or healthy person. Everyone is different. Thus, each person's daily water requirements will vary.

It is a widespread misunderstanding that everyone should drink eight glasses of water daily.

The kidneys control the volume and makeup of body fluids. Fundamental regulatory mechanisms involving the kidneys are responsible for regulating volume, sodium and potassium concentrations, and pH of body fluids.

The kidneys are the primary site of controlled water excretion. The skin, lungs, and feces also contribute to water loss, approximately a liter daily. Understanding how sodium and water control work

The Role of Functional Kidneys in Preventing Failure

together to protect the body from potential changes in the volume and osmolality of physiological fluids is crucial.

Disorders such as dehydration, blood loss, salt consumption, and plain water overconsumption impact this balance. Water balance is established in the body by ensuring that the amount of water taken in through food and drink (and produced by metabolism) balances the amount of water expelled. The behavioral processes that control consumption include salt and thirst desires.

The abrupt onset of acute renal failure and its frequent reversibility

Accidents, injuries, illnesses, infections, shock, and drug or poison consumption are a few causes. The kidneys stop making urine when they are injured. As poisons accumulate in the bloodstream, the patient becomes confused, unconscious, and bloated.

Kidney function could improve with treatment, while chronic kidney failure occurs gradually and typically cannot be reversed. A diet, hydration restrictions, and temporary dialysis are prescribed to patients with acute renal failure until their kidneys have healed.

Dialysis is typically necessary if the disease has advanced and the kidneys no longer function at 10 to 15 percent of normal levels. Even though dialysis carries out some of the activities of healthy kidneys, it does not treat kidney disease. The patient will typically require kidney transplantation or dialysis for the remainder of their life.

Acute kidney injury (AKI) within the first 48 hours following the occurrence causes serum creatinine to rise by 0.3 percent. Blood urea nitrogen (BUN) also increases, and glomerular filtration rate (GFR) rapidly falls within hours to days.

Are condiments like salt resulting in hypertension and sugar in diabetes mellitus behind acute or chronic kidney failure?

High blood sugar resulting from diabetes leads to damaged blood vessels in the kidney. Each kidney consists of millions of tiny filters known as nephrons. As a result, nephrons are also affected and cease to function as they should. Additionally, diabetes may lead to high blood pressure (hypertension). Both hypertension and diabetes mellitus are some of the significant risk factors for chronic kidney failure. These two factors account for 70 percent of end-stage kidney disease cases.

Condiments like salt (sodium) increase blood pressure, so a low-salt diet is recommended for all those suffering from hypertension. The recommended intake is a maximum of 2400 mg to 3000 mg. To make it easier to understand, any food with more than 400 mg of sodium per serving falls under the category of high sodium. Salt intake is associated with impaired kidney function among the general population, especially those with diabetes mellitus and hypertension. Salt intake is linked to developing chronic kidney disease and affects blood pressure. It also affects the estimated

The Role of Functional Kidneys in Preventing Failure

glomerular filtration rate (eGFR). eGFR measures the effectiveness of the kidneys. It offers an estimated number, considering factors such as age, race, body type, and more.

What are the effects of medications containing salt compounds given to patients with low blood pressure, aside from NaCl saline bags?

Providing healthy blood pressure will ensure adequate oxygen supply to the brain tissue. Medications containing salt cause your blood volume to expand by ensuring fluid retention in the venous circulatory system, thereby preventing blood pressure from dropping. This will help ensure there are no episodes of syncope.

Tips to prevent kidney failure

Kidneys can be kept healthy by addressing risk factors. By managing risk factors, all individuals can prevent the onset of chronic kidney disease and other associated complications. According to the CDC, the following tips help contain the threat of CKD:

- Losing weight if you are obese
- Being physically active as it helps control blood sugar levels
- Quitting smoking
- Getting checked regularly to ensure your kidney is healthy
- Taking medications as prescribed and directed by the doctor

- Maintaining blood pressure below 140/90
- Staying in the recommended blood sugar range for those who have diabetes
- Not exceeding the target cholesterol range
- Consuming foods containing less salt
- Eating a diet rich in fruits and vegetables

How to manage CKD

If you are already suffering from CKD, then you need to implement the following changes:

- Healthy eating by conforming to a renal diet as proposed by a dietician
- Taking proper medications
- Avoiding medications and kidney infections that may cause harm to the kidneys. Medications that need to be avoided include over-the-counter pain medications such as ibuprofen and naproxen, and certain antibiotics
- Avoiding dyes used for making organs or blood vessels visible on X-rays and other imaging tests

Is stem cell therapy for kidney failure an excellent alternative to a kidney transplant?

Stem cell therapy can benefit patients suffering from moderate to

The Role of Functional Kidneys in Preventing Failure

late or terminal stage renal failure by removing the need for dialysis or reducing the frequency of dialysis. Stem cell treatment can repair kidney damage and prevent additional harm to renal function in patients with early-stage renal failure or kidney disease. Our functional regenerative medical therapies employing improved renal stem cells allow patients the certainty that their kidneys will not deteriorate or cause other concerns such as heart disease (heart attacks), pancreatic failure (diabetic nephropathy), and other complications.[10]

"Although it is challenging to regenerate the kidney in vitro completely, recent developments in the field of stem cells have made it possible to create organoids in vitro. When creating new kidney tissues for transplantation, induced pluripotent stem cells are the most significant source because they can potentially come from patients and be utilized as a renal replacement therapy without immunosuppression. Based on research, when creating fresh kidney tissues for transplantation, induced pluripotent stem cells are the ideal source because they can potentially come from patients and be utilized as a renal replacement therapy without immunosuppression."[11]

---

[10] https://stemcellthailand.org/therapies/renal-failure-kidney-disease/
[11] https://www.healthcentral.com/article/collagen-supplements-and-kidneys

2:
Introduction to Dialysis: Process, Purpose, and People

Albumin as an Indicator of Diseases Beyond Nutritional Deficiency in Adults

Understanding the complexities of kidney health begins with recognizing critical biomarkers that reveal underlying pathological processes. Among these, **serum albumin** stands out not only as a marker of nutritional status but also as a powerful prognostic indicator for a range of chronic and acute conditions, especially in individuals with compromised renal function.

Traditionally, low albumin levels have been associated with protein-energy malnutrition. However, emerging clinical evidence underscores that hypoalbuminemia in adults, particularly in patients undergoing dialysis, is more often linked to inflammation, infection, fluid overload, and chronic disease progression than to dietary insufficiency alone.

In patients with chronic kidney disease (CKD) or end-stage renal disease (ESRD), serum albumin levels below 3.5 g/dL are frequently observed and strongly correlated with:

- Increased mortality risk

- Cardiovascular events
- Poor wound healing
- Prolonged hospitalization

This has led nephrologists and clinicians to consider albumin a negative acute-phase reactant, meaning its levels decrease in response to systemic inflammation, oxidative stress, or infection, conditions commonly seen in CKD and dialysis patients.

Ferritin, another key biomarker, adds further depth to this assessment. While typically used to evaluate iron stores, elevated ferritin levels in CKD patients often reflect chronic inflammation rather than iron sufficiency, especially when accompanied by normal or elevated transferrin saturation (TSAT).

Key considerations for interpreting albumin in CKD include:

- Persistent hypoalbuminemia may signal underlying inflammatory states such as infections, autoimmune diseases, or malignancies.
- Overhydration or dilutional states common in dialysis patients can falsely lower measured albumin levels.
- Liver dysfunction, protein-losing enteropathy, or nephrotic syndrome may also contribute to low albumin and should be ruled out accordingly.

Clinical Implications:

Monitoring albumin levels over time, alongside markers like C-reactive protein (CRP), ferritin, and TSAT, allows for a more nuanced understanding of patient status. This supports timely interventions, such as anti-inflammatory treatment, infection control, fluid management, or nutritional support tailored to the underlying cause rather than focusing solely on protein intake.

In conclusion, while albumin remains an important nutritional marker, it has evolved into a broader indicator of disease severity, systemic inflammation, and clinical outcomes in adults, especially those with kidney-related conditions. Recognizing its multifactorial implications can significantly enhance patient management and prognosis.

Albumin: More Than a Marker of Nutrition

Albumin, a vital protein found in blood plasma, is traditionally used to assess liver and kidney function. Although low albumin levels are often associated with kidney disease, they can also point to other serious conditions, such as liver disease, infections, or systemic inflammation. In some cases, symptoms like chronic diarrhea or dehydration may also lower albumin levels.

When albumin levels are found to be low, physicians do not simply attribute it to poor nutrition. Instead, they pursue a deeper investigation, often ordering comprehensive blood and urine tests to determine the root cause. While nutritional deficiencies, such as insufficient protein intake, can certainly affect albumin levels, these deviations may signal far more complex medical concerns that require prompt and thorough evaluation.

Low albumin may indicate kidney dysfunction, especially when paired with symptoms such as:

- Loss of appetite
- Fatigue
- Trouble concentrating
- Frequent urination
- Itchy or dry skin
- Muscle cramps
- General weakness
- Nausea or vomiting
- Swelling in the face, ankles, or feet
- Noticeable changes in urine

These warning signs, combined with diagnostic markers, can help guide timely intervention and improve patient outcomes.

Ferritin and Its Hidden Influence on Kidney Health

Ferritin, a protein responsible for storing iron in the blood, plays a more dynamic role in kidney health than is commonly recognized. It not only reflects iron reserves but also serves as a protective agent for the kidneys following injury by regulating iron distribution and minimizing oxidative stress.

A ferritin test helps evaluate whether your iron stores are adequate. Low ferritin levels typically point to iron deficiency, but elevated levels may reveal more concerning trends. In the context of chronic kidney disease, particularly glomerular disorders and proteinuria, high ferritin can signal progressive dysfunction.

Ferritin as an Inflammation Indicator

Ferritin also functions as a biomarker of inflammation, offering insights that go beyond iron balance. In individuals with obesity, for example, high ferritin levels may uncover hidden, low-grade inflammation that would otherwise go undetected. During infection or acute illness, ferritin levels often rise as part of the immune response. This elevation helps the body by reducing iron availability to harmful bacteria, supporting immune function, and limiting oxidative damage caused by free radicals.

It is worth noting, however, that not every fluctuation in ferritin requires clinical intervention. Around five percent of healthy individuals may have levels outside the typical range without any underlying disease. In such cases, context and additional diagnostic findings are essential to determine whether further investigation or treatment is needed.

Managing a Vegan Protein Diet for CKD and Dialysis Patients

Adopting a plant-based diet can be a powerful tool for individuals living with chronic kidney disease (CKD), offering benefits that extend far beyond kidney function. This dietary approach can help slow disease progression, reduce inflammation, and support the management of common comorbidities such as type 2 diabetes, hypertension, and cardiovascular disease. Replacing red and processed meats with plant-derived protein alternatives is particularly effective in reducing the kidney's metabolic burden and minimizing further damage.

The Role of Plant-Based Nutrition in CKD

Extensive research highlights the protective effects of whole grains, fruits, vegetables, legumes, and nuts in preserving renal function. These foods are rich in antioxidants, fiber, and phytochemicals that support systemic health. Importantly, a plant-based diet does not require the complete elimination of animal products but rather encourages a balanced shift toward more sustainable, kidney-friendly protein sources.

For individuals already following vegetarian or vegan diets, a CKD or dialysis diagnosis does not mandate a switch to animal-based proteins. With proper planning, a vegan diet can provide adequate nutrition, support metabolic stability, and align with the patient's ethical or cultural values.

Protein Considerations for Dialysis Patients

Patients on dialysis require higher protein intake due to the loss of amino acids and proteins during treatment. However, this increase must be carefully balanced with the need to manage phosphorus, potassium, and sodium levels.

Recommended vegan protein sources for dialysis patients include:

- Tofu and tempeh: Low in potassium and phosphorus (especially when prepared with care).

- Lentils, chickpeas, and black beans: Rich in protein, but may require portion control or phosphate binders.

- Quinoa, amaranth, and buckwheat: High-quality plant proteins with a complete amino acid profile.

- Seitan and plant-based meat substitutes: Useful for variety, though patients should monitor sodium content.

- Nuts and seeds (in moderation): Provide healthy fats and protein but should be portioned due to phosphorus content.

Specialized vegan renal protein supplements, low in potassium, phosphorus, and artificial sweeteners, can also be used to meet protein needs without compromising mineral balance.

Introduction to Dialysis: Process, Purpose, and People

Nutritional Support and Supplementation

In addition to protein, dialysis patients may require caloric supplementation to prevent malnutrition, particularly in cases of low appetite or unintentional weight loss. This can include:

- Plant-based oils (e.g., olive, flaxseed)
- Smoothies made with renal-safe ingredients
- Nutrient-dense snacks tailored to individual lab values

To manage hyperkalemia, patients may require a low-potassium dialysate, and food preparation techniques such as leaching vegetables or choosing lower-potassium produce (e.g., apples, berries, cabbage) become critical.

Benefits of a Plant-Forward Approach

A thoughtful, plant-forward renal diet has been shown to:

- Slow glomerular filtration rate (GFR) decline
- Reduce cyst growth in conditions like polycystic kidney disease (PKD)
- Improve lipid profiles and insulin sensitivity
- Lower systemic inflammation and acidosis

In earlier stages of CKD, protein restriction is often emphasized to minimize nitrogenous waste buildup. However, once dialysis begins, protein requirements increase significantly, typically to 1.2

g/kg/day or more, depending on modality and clinical status.

Collagen-Based Protein in Dialysis and Kidney Transplant Patients

Collagen, the most abundant protein in the human body, plays an integral role in maintaining the strength, structure, and elasticity of connective tissues, supporting muscles, ligaments, tendons, and skin. As we age, collagen production gradually declines, beginning in our twenties and decreasing by approximately one percent each year. Lifestyle factors like poor sleep, excessive alcohol use, physical inactivity, and sun exposure can accelerate this decline.

Collagen supplements have surged in popularity for their potential benefits in joint and skin health. However, for patients with kidney disease or those recovering from a kidney transplant, caution is critical. According to Dr. David P. Selzer, a nephrologist at NYU Langone Medical Associates, many collagen products contain hydroxyproline, an amino acid that is metabolized into oxalate. The body cannot break down oxalate further, and excess amounts can lead to kidney stone formation or worsen existing kidney problems.

Before incorporating collagen supplements into a renal diet, patients should consult their healthcare team to evaluate risks and identify safer alternatives if necessary.

Introduction to Dialysis: Process, Purpose, and People

Central Venous Catheters (CVCs) and Infection Risks

Central venous catheters (CVCs) are a lifeline for many patients receiving dialysis, chemotherapy, or other critical treatments. However, they carry a high risk of bloodstream infections, which are among the most serious hospital-acquired complications. These infections are linked to increased morbidity, extended hospital stays, and higher healthcare costs.

Several factors influence infection risk, including the type of organism involved, the patient's immune status, and the timeliness of diagnosis and intervention. The growing use of immunosuppressive medications has increased susceptibility to opportunistic infections, including rare but dangerous pathogens such as filamentous fungi.

A clinical example illustrates the risk: a 13-year-old undergoing treatment for acute lymphoblastic leukemia was hospitalized with a fever of unknown origin. To pinpoint the source of infection, blood samples were taken from both the central catheter and a peripheral vein. This approach helped identify the infection site and determine the appropriate course of treatment.

Gram-negative organisms cause 20 to 30 percent of catheter-related bloodstream infections (CRBSIs), while gram-positive bacteria are responsible for 40 to 80 percent. The most common pathogens include coagulase-negative staphylococci, *Staphylococcus aureus*, and *Enterococcus*. Methicillin-resistant staphylococci are also frequently identified.

Factors Contributing to Pathogen Inoculation

Central line-associated bloodstream infections (CLABSIs) result in thousands of deaths annually and impose billions of dollars in healthcare costs, despite being largely preventable. The CDC provides evidence-based recommendations and resources to reduce the incidence of CLABSIs.

The Role of Hand Hygiene

Since CVCs account for nearly 90 percent of catheter-related infections, strict hygiene practices are crucial. These catheters also play a vital role in hemodynamic monitoring, making infection control even more important. Hand hygiene is widely acknowledged as the most effective and economical strategy to combat infections.

The World Health Organization outlines "Five Moments for Hand Hygiene" that healthcare professionals must follow:

- Before touching a patient
- Before performing a clean or aseptic procedure
- After exposure to bodily fluids
- After touching a patient
- After touching patient surroundings

Introduction to Dialysis: Process, Purpose, and People

Using an alcohol-based hand sanitizer at each of these critical moments significantly reduces infection risks.

CVC Infection Rates in the United States

Between 2008 and 2013, the U.S. saw a 46 percent decrease in CLABSIs in hospitals. Nevertheless, approximately 30,100 CLABSIs still occur annually in intensive care units and other hospital wards.

Prevention programs and continued nursing education remain essential to further reduce infection rates and enhance patient safety.

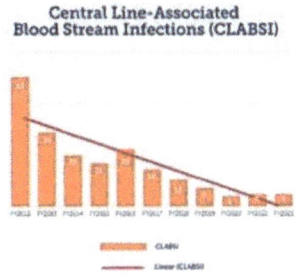

Image of CLABSI

Use of Povidone Iodine and Alcohol Prep to Kill Bacteria, Fungi, Mycobacteria, and Viruses

Over the past six decades, povidone iodine (PVP-I) formulations have played a vital role in reducing the spread and impact of infectious diseases. PVP-I is known for its broad-spectrum antimicrobial properties, offering potent antiviral, antibacterial, and antifungal effects.

In contrast to alcohol, which leaves many bacteria active after disinfection, povidone iodine provides more comprehensive protection. Its rapid and substantial disinfecting action is particularly effective in maintaining the sterility of central venous catheters (CVCs), helping prevent complications during medical procedures.

Cooling Dialysate Solution to Prevent Fungal and Microbial Growth

Controlling the temperature of dialysate solutions during hemodialysis is crucial for preventing heat buildup and maintaining patient safety. Cooling the dialysate induces peripheral vasoconstriction, which helps prevent intradialytic hypotension, a common complication that can interrupt treatment and require medical intervention.

Maintaining a stable body temperature helps ensure the efficiency of the dialysis process. It also minimizes moisture accumulation, which is a key factor in the growth of fungi and microorganisms. The standard dialysate temperature used for long-term hemodialysis patients is 37°C (98.6°F), a level that balances patient comfort with clinical efficacy.

Preventing Fungal Growth from High-Sugar GT Supplements

Candida infections, particularly those caused by *Candida albicans*, thrive in environments where glucose levels are elevated, making dietary sugar intake a significant factor in the onset and persistence of fungal overgrowth. Individuals with diabetes, compromised immunity, or those undergoing gastrointestinal therapy (GT) using high-sugar nutritional supplements are particularly at risk.

GT supplements, especially those used in tube feeding or post-surgical recovery, may contain high levels of glucose, maltodextrin, or other rapidly absorbed carbohydrates, which can disrupt the balance of gut flora. These conditions create an ideal environment for yeast proliferation, particularly in the oral cavity, gastrointestinal tract, or genitourinary system.

Risk Factors for Fungal Overgrowth

- High intake of sugar or refined carbohydrates
- Use of broad-spectrum antibiotics
- Diabetes mellitus with poor glycemic control
- Use of corticosteroids or immunosuppressants
- Prolonged use of high-sugar GT supplements
- Oral or enteral feeding tubes without adequate hygiene

Preventive Strategies

1. **Opt for Low-Sugar GT Supplements:**

   Choose enteral nutrition formulas designed for glycemic control or renal health. These often have reduced sugar content and are better suited for patients prone to infections or metabolic imbalance.

2. **Monitor and Control Blood Glucose:**

   Maintaining **tight glycemic control** reduces the risk of candida overgrowth, especially in diabetic or ICU patients receiving nutrition through GT.

3. **Support Gut Microbiota:**

   Incorporating **probiotics**, such as *Lactobacillus rhamnosus* or *Saccharomyces boulardii*, under medical supervision can help restore healthy microbial balance and inhibit fungal colonization.

4. **Practice Proper Tube Hygiene:**

   Regular cleaning of feeding tubes and oral care is critical. Residual formula can act as a breeding ground for pathogens if not cleaned adequately.

5. **Consider Antifungal Prophylaxis in High-Risk Patients:**

   In patients with recurrent fungal infections or

immunocompromised states, short-term antifungal prophylaxis may be considered under medical advice.

Treatment Approaches

When fungal infections occur, they can manifest as **oral thrush, esophagitis, skin rashes, vaginal candidiasis**, or **systemic infections** in severe cases. Treatment options include:

- **Mild to Moderate Infections:**
    - *Oral fluconazole (Diflucan)*: A single 150 mg dose is often effective for uncomplicated cases such as vaginal candidiasis.
    - *Topical antifungals:* Butoconazole (Gynazole), clotrimazole, or miconazole for localized infections.
- **Severe or Recurrent Infections:**
    - Extended courses of **oral or intravenous antifungals**, such as fluconazole, itraconazole, or amphotericin B, may be required.
    - **Diagnostic testing**, including fungal cultures or sensitivity testing, helps guide treatment in resistant cases.
- **Adjunctive Measures:**
    - Elimination or reduction of high-sugar supplements

- Reassessment of nutritional needs and GT formulation
- Improved glycemic control and immune support

Maintaining Baseline Blood Pressure in Hemodialysis Patients

Baseline blood pressure (BP) serves as a critical marker for evaluating the effectiveness of antihypertensive therapy. In patients with end-stage renal disease, elevated blood pressure is common and contributes significantly to cardiovascular complications.

Maintaining blood pressure near a patient's baseline is essential to prolong life expectancy among those on hemodialysis. Uncontrolled hypertension remains a significant challenge in these patients, with sodium and fluid retention being the primary culprits.

Non-pharmacologic approaches to managing BP include individualized dialysate sodium prescriptions and gradual dry-weight reduction. These strategies are crucial for reducing the burden of hypertension and achieving BP targets, ultimately improving patient outcomes during dialysis.

Time Management in Hemodialysis

Hemodialysis can be administered either in a clinical center or at home. In-center treatments are usually scheduled three times a week, with each session lasting three to four hours. Proper planning is essential, as these sessions are typically set in advance and require

Introduction to Dialysis: Process, Purpose, and People

coordination with medical staff.

Home dialysis offers greater flexibility. Conventional home hemodialysis follows a similar schedule to in-center treatment, three or more sessions a week, each lasting several hours. Short daily home hemodialysis involves more frequent sessions (five to seven times weekly), but each treatment lasts only two hours. Another option, nocturnal hemodialysis, is performed at night while the patient sleeps and typically lasts six to eight hours, up to six nights per week or every other night as prescribed.

Short daily hemodialysis offers numerous advantages. It reduces the need for medications to manage blood pressure, anemia, and phosphorus levels. Patients often report better nerve function, reduced restless leg syndrome, improved sleep, and more energy for daily activities. These benefits translate into a better quality of life and fewer hospitalizations.

Studies show that patients receiving fewer hours of dialysis per session tend to have higher systolic blood pressure. By contrast, extending dialysis to four hours per session can lead to better blood pressure control, even with fewer weekly sessions. This highlights the importance of adequate dialysis time for managing hypertension and improving long-term outcomes.

Fungal growth thrives at room temperatures, particularly around 25°C. As temperatures rise, fungal development significantly decreases. However, fungal contamination in dialysate solutions poses a serious threat to dialysis patients, who already have compromised immune systems.

Hemodialysis, the primary treatment for patients with end-stage renal disease, is typically conducted three times a week, with sessions lasting between three and four hours depending on the individual's clinical condition. During each session, large volumes of water are used to produce the dialysate and in the reuse of dialyzers. On average, a dialysis patient is exposed to approximately 400 liters of water weekly. This high exposure underscores the critical importance of maintaining exceptional water quality to minimize health risks, particularly fungal contamination, which could lead to systemic infections and treatment complications.

Hypotension in Dialysis Patients: Causes and Treatment

Hypotension during dialysis, commonly referred to as dialysis-induced hypotension, occurs due to the body's inadequate cardiovascular response to a rapid decrease in blood volume. This fluid removal, while necessary for treatment, reduces cardiac filling and challenges the body's ability to maintain stable blood pressure.

The condition is influenced by both patient-related and dialysis-related factors, including preexisting cardiovascular health and the rate at which fluid is removed. As a result, many patients experience hypotension during sessions. Prompt treatment involves intravenous

Introduction to Dialysis: Process, Purpose, and People

fluid replacement to quickly restore blood volume and stabilize the patient, allowing them to safely complete the session and leave the dialysis unit.

Maintaining Fluid Balance Through Dry Weight

Effective dialysis depends on precise fluid volume and hemodynamic management. One clinical method used to achieve this is the "dry weight" approach, defined as the patient's weight when excess fluid has been removed, without causing hypotension or dehydration. Proper salt and water homeostasis is essential for the cardiovascular health of dialysis patients.

The importance of fluid management is closely tied to the issue of hypotension. Cardiovascular filling must be preserved during treatment, and achieving this requires a more sophisticated and individualized strategy.

Accurate assessment and monitoring of fluid status involve four key components:

- Clinical assessment
- Non-invasive tools, such as blood volume monitoring
- Cardiac biomarkers
- Algorithms and sodium modeling for mass transfer estimation

Managing fluid and sodium levels in dialysis patients is a delicate and essential process. Achieving this balance involves more than just removing excess fluid, it requires a strategic and personalized approach. Ultrafiltration and dialysate sodium adjustments are only part of the equation. Equally important is the control of dietary salt intake and fluid consumption between dialysis sessions, both of which play critical roles in maintaining overall health and preventing complications.

Advancements in technology have revolutionized how clinicians approach fluid management. Tools such as biosensors, real-time feedback control systems, and advanced data analytics allow for tailored treatment plans that respond to each patient's unique physiology. While the traditional "dry weight" guideline offers a helpful clinical baseline, it does not fully address the intricate cardiovascular dynamics involved. For this reason, a broader, more integrated strategy is needed, one that blends fluid and hemodynamic management into a single, cohesive framework.

Hemodynamic stability is vital. True fluid balance, or euvolemia, is not simply about removing enough fluid, it involves harmonizing the body's total fluid volume with cardiovascular function and metabolic needs. Achieving euvolemia requires constant assessment and adjustment. When managed effectively, it leads to improved treatment outcomes and supports the long-term health of dialysis patients.

Introduction to Dialysis: Process, Purpose, and People

Fluid overload and dehydration both pose serious risks. Edema, shortness of breath, elevated blood pressure, and cardiac strain are common consequences of poor fluid control. Because every patient is different, the allowable fluid intake must be carefully determined based on several factors. These include the patient's residual kidney function, urine output, comorbidities, nutritional status, and individual tolerance to fluid shifts.

One of the most important tools in assessing fluid balance is weight monitoring. By weighing patients before and after dialysis sessions, healthcare teams can accurately calculate the volume of fluid removed. Significant weight gains between sessions often signal fluid retention, prompting the need for stricter fluid intake limits and recalibrated ultrafiltration goals.

The ultrafiltration rate is a key parameter. It dictates how much fluid is extracted during each session and must be closely monitored to avoid complications such as intradialytic hypotension or muscle cramping. When set appropriately, it helps maintain euvolemia while minimizing patient discomfort and cardiovascular stress.

Effective fluid management is not just a clinical responsibility, it is a shared commitment between patients and their healthcare teams. Patient engagement, education, and open dialogue are vital components. When patients understand their fluid restrictions and the importance of treatment adherence, they are more likely to participate actively in their care. This collaboration empowers patients, fosters trust, and leads to better health outcomes.

In summary, achieving and maintaining fluid balance in dialysis patients demands a multifaceted and personalized strategy. It involves careful weight monitoring, precise ultrafiltration, dietary guidance, and continuous clinical evaluation. By embracing advanced technology and encouraging patient participation, healthcare providers can create individualized care plans that protect cardiovascular health, enhance quality of life, and reduce the risks associated with fluid imbalances.

3:
Uncovering the Root Causes of Dialysis Needs

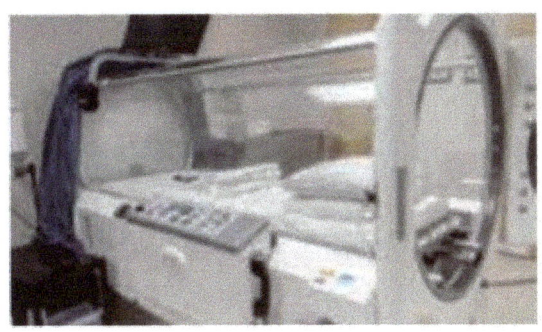

Hyperbaric Oxygen Therapy: A Vital Adjunct for Dialysis Patients with Severe Anemia

Hyperbaric oxygen therapy (HBOT) is an advanced medical treatment that involves breathing 100 percent oxygen in a specially designed pressurized chamber. While commonly used to treat conditions such as brain abscesses, arterial gas embolism, and chronic wounds, HBOT is gaining attention for its potential role in improving outcomes for patients undergoing dialysis, especially those struggling with severe anemia.

In the context of dialysis, severe anemia presents a critical challenge. Reduced red blood cell count limits oxygen delivery to tissues, exacerbating fatigue, impairing cognitive function, and increasing cardiovascular risk. HBOT offers a unique solution by significantly increasing the amount of oxygen dissolved in the plasma, known as the partial pressure of dissolved oxygen. Unlike traditional oxygen therapies that rely on hemoglobin, HBOT bypasses this limitation, delivering oxygen directly to oxygen-deprived tissues without placing additional strain on the heart or lungs.

Moreover, HBOT fosters a healing environment at the cellular level. It stimulates the mobilization of peripheral progenitor cells, essential agents of tissue repair and regeneration, and enhances angiogenesis, the formation of new blood vessels. This process helps reverse renal hypoxia, improve microcirculation, and support overall organ function, making it particularly beneficial for dialysis patients with compromised oxygenation and chronic inflammation.

Who Should Not Undergo Hyperbaric Oxygen Therapy (HBOT)?

Despite its well-documented therapeutic benefits in conditions such as diabetic foot ulcers, radiation injury, and carbon monoxide poisoning, Hyperbaric Oxygen Therapy (HBOT) is not appropriate for all individuals. Certain medical conditions, physiological risks, and psychological factors can make HBOT potentially dangerous or ineffective. Comprehensive medical screening is essential to identify contraindications and ensure patient safety.

Uncovering the Root Causes of Dialysis Needs

Absolute Contraindications

These are conditions in which HBOT should not be administered under any circumstances:

- **Untreated Pneumothorax:**

    The presence of free air in the pleural cavity can expand under pressure, increasing the risk of a **tension pneumothorax**, which may be fatal without immediate intervention.

Relative Contraindications

These conditions may not entirely exclude a patient from HBOT, but they require **careful evaluation and risk-benefit analysis** by a qualified physician:

- **Chronic Obstructive Pulmonary Disease (COPD) with Air Trapping or Bullae:**

    COPD patients may have fragile lung tissue and air pockets (blebs or bullae) that increase the risk of **barotrauma**, including **lung rupture or pneumothorax**, when exposed to high-pressure environments.

- **Recent Thoracic or Ear Surgery:**

    Surgical changes in chest or middle ear anatomy can make it difficult to equalize pressure, increasing the risk of **barotrauma** or **surgical site complications**.

- **Upper Respiratory Infections or Sinus Congestion:**

    These can prevent proper ear or sinus pressure equalization, leading to **painful barotrauma or eardrum rupture.**

- **Severe Claustrophobia or Anxiety Disorders:**

    Patients who experience **panic attacks or distress in enclosed spaces** may not tolerate the therapy chamber without sedation or behavioral therapy.

- **Fever or Uncontrolled Seizure Disorders:**

    Elevated body temperature or a history of seizures increases the risk of **oxygen toxicity seizures**, a known but rare complication of HBOT.

- **Pregnancy (in certain cases):**

    While HBOT is sometimes used in pregnant women (e.g., for carbon monoxide poisoning), it is generally avoided unless the **benefit clearly outweighs the risk** to the fetus.

- **Severe Congestive Heart Failure or Uncontrolled Hypertension:**

    The increased oxygen pressure can lead to **hemodynamic shifts** that may worsen cardiovascular instability.

- **Use of Certain Medications:**

    Some drugs (e.g., **doxorubicin, cisplatin, disulfiram**) can interact adversely with hyperbaric oxygen, increasing the risk of toxicity.

- **History of Ear Barotrauma or Tympanic Membrane Rupture:**
Inability to equalize middle ear pressure may result in **pain or further damage** during therapy.

Potential Risks of HBOT

Even in eligible patients, the following risks must be discussed:

- Oxygen toxicity (CNS or pulmonary)
- Barotrauma to ears, sinuses, or lungs
- Temporary visual changes (myopia)
- Hypoglycemia in diabetic patients (due to increased metabolism during treatment)
- Fire hazard in the chamber (strict safety protocols are essential)

Anemia and Hyperbaric oxygen therapy

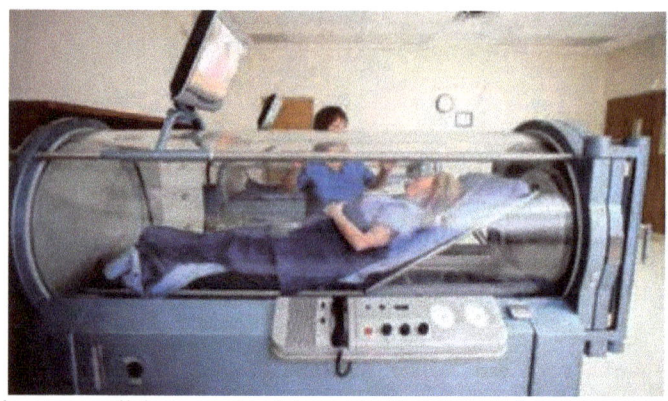

Anemia, a condition marked by a deficiency of red blood cells or hemoglobin, severely impairs the blood's ability to transport oxygen. This leads to symptoms such as fatigue, pallor, weakness, and in severe cases, shock. Causes of anemia include significant blood loss, impaired red blood cell production in the bone marrow, and red blood cell destruction due to underlying disease.

HBOT directly addresses the oxygen deficiency in anemic patients by delivering oxygen more efficiently to vital organs, offering a critical lifeline in managing this life-threatening condition.

Treating Gangrene with HBOT

In addition to anemia, HBOT is highly effective in treating gangrene. It accelerates healing in cases of carbon monoxide poisoning, non-healing wounds, and gangrenous tissues. The therapy delivers concentrated oxygen to deprived tissues, reducing infection risks and supporting recovery. While other treatments for gangrene, like antibiotics and surgery, are essential, early diagnosis and the addition of HBOT significantly improve outcomes.

HBOT for Infections

HBOT is beneficial for treating chronic and severe infections such as necrotizing fasciitis and osteomyelitis. It also supports the management of infective endocarditis and soft tissue infections by restoring oxygen to areas where blood supply has been compromised.

Supporting Brain Injury Recovery

Hyperbaric oxygen therapy is gaining attention for its potential to aid recovery from chronic traumatic brain injury (TBI). TBI remains one of the leading causes of injury-related death in the United States, and HBOT may help improve symptoms long term by enhancing oxygen delivery to damaged brain tissue.

Supplementing Anemia Medications in Dialysis Patients

Dialysis patients often rely on medications such as Mircera, Aranesp, and other erythropoiesis-stimulating agents (ESAs) to manage anemia. However, these drugs can cause serious side effects. HBOT offers a supportive therapy that may reduce dependence on such medications.

Iron, a vital mineral for oxygen transport and overall health, also plays a critical role. It helps produce myoglobin for muscle oxygenation, strengthens the immune system, supports gastrointestinal function, regulates body temperature, and boosts energy levels. Iron deficiency can result in symptoms such as heart palpitations, fatigue, breathlessness, and pale skin.

In women, especially during adolescence and pregnancy, the need for iron increases due to menstrual blood loss and fetal development demands. Adequate iron levels are also linked to cognitive function, focus, memory, and even hair health. Symptoms such as fatigue, low energy, and heavy menstrual cycles often indicate a need for iron supplementation.

In conclusion, hyperbaric oxygen therapy represents a promising adjunct to traditional dialysis and anemia treatments. When used thoughtfully and in the right clinical context, it can improve oxygen delivery, reduce complications, and enhance the overall quality of life for patients with complex, interrelated conditions.

Maintaining the right balance of iron is critical, as both deficiency and excess can adversely affect the body. Iron levels directly influence blood pressure regulation. While iron supplements paired with dietary sources generally do not show a significant effect on blood pressure, extremely high doses, particularly in children, can cause dangerously low blood pressure and, in severe cases, result in death.

On the other hand, iron supplementation in children born with low birth weight has been shown to help prevent the onset of hypertension in both childhood and later adulthood. These supplements regulate iron levels, helping to stabilize red blood cell concentration and prevent pulmonary-related blood pressure issues.

For dialysis patients, maintaining a balance between water and fiber intake is especially important when taking iron supplements. Without proper hydration and fiber, side effects such as stomach pain and constipation are common. Moreover, increasing fiber intake helps reduce serum uremic toxins, which accumulate due to kidney dysfunction.

Dialysis patients should be encouraged to eat more fiber-rich foods, such as pulses, lentils, whole grains, fruits, and vegetables. To manage both fiber and fluid effectively, patients can benefit from reducing salt intake. Excess salt leads the body to retain water, increasing thirst and complicating fluid management.

A practical approach to balance is dividing fiber and fluid intake into smaller, manageable portions throughout the day. For example, taking several ounces of water with each fiber-rich meal or snack can improve digestion and enhance nutrient absorption without overloading the system.

Erythropoiesis-stimulating agents (ESAs) are medications that stimulate the bone marrow to produce more red blood cells. These drugs are particularly useful in treating anemia caused by chronic kidney disease and certain chemotherapy regimens. ESAs also help reduce the need for blood transfusions, especially in patients undergoing major surgeries.

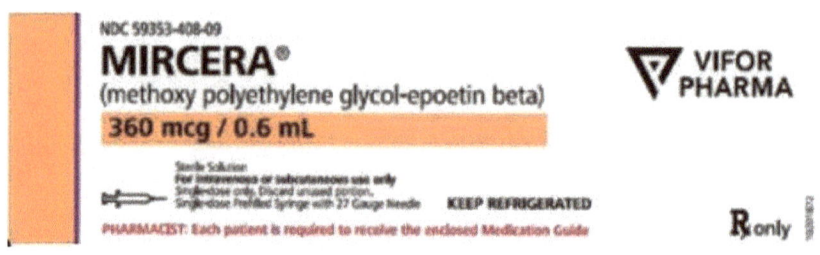

Mircera is an ESA used to treat anemia stemming from chronic kidney disease in adults, whether or not they require dialysis. However, it has many unpleasant side effects, such as headaches, diarrhea, body aches, and vomiting.

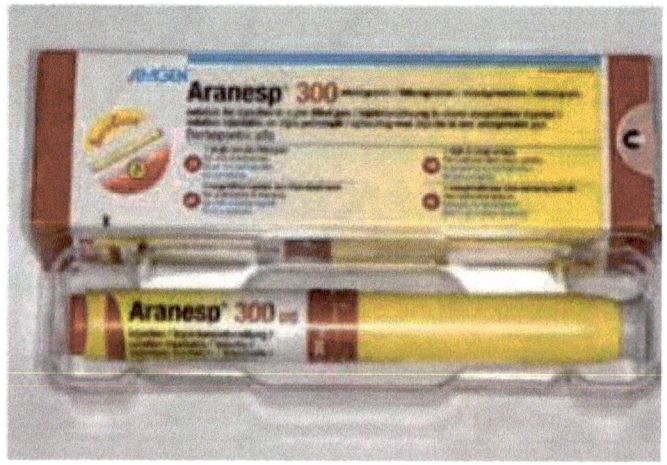

Aranesp is another medication used to treat anemia. It, too, has many unpleasant side effects, such as cough and shortness of breath, and it can cause low blood pressure during dialysis.

Hyperbaric oxygen therapy is helpful, as it can supplement these medications that have significant side effects.

Relationship Between UTIs and Diabetes

UTIs, or urinary tract infections, occur when bacteria, most commonly *Escherichia coli* (E. coli), from the skin or rectum enter the urethra and multiply within the urinary tract. These infections can affect different parts of the urinary system, including the urethra (urethritis), bladder (cystitis), and kidneys (pyelonephritis). Among these, bladder infections (cystitis) are the most common form.

People with diabetes are at a higher risk of developing UTIs for several reasons:

1. **Weakened Immune System**: Chronic high blood sugar levels can impair the body's immune response, making it harder to fight off infections, including UTIs.

2. **High Glucose in Urine**: Elevated glucose levels in urine create an ideal environment for bacteria to grow, increasing the risk of infection.

3. **Nerve Damage (Autonomic Neuropathy)**: Diabetes-related nerve damage can affect bladder function, leading to incomplete emptying of the bladder. This urinary retention allows bacteria to multiply, increasing the likelihood of a

UTI.

4. **Poor Circulation**: Reduced blood flow caused by diabetes can slow down the body's ability to heal and fight infections effectively.

5. **Frequent UTIs**: Individuals with diabetes may experience more frequent or recurrent UTIs, and these infections may be more severe or harder to treat.

6. **Asymptomatic Infections**: Diabetic patients, especially women, may have asymptomatic bacteriuria (bacteria in the urine without symptoms), which can progress to more serious infections if untreated.

7. **Risk of Complications**: UTIs in people with diabetes are more likely to lead to complications such as kidney infections (pyelonephritis), sepsis, or even renal abscesses if not promptly and adequately managed.

Because of these factors, it is crucial for individuals with diabetes to

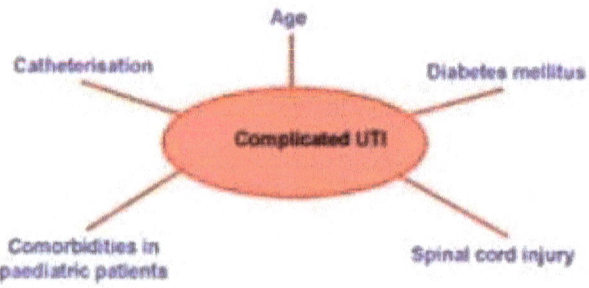

manage their blood sugar levels, practice good hygiene, and seek medical attention if they experience symptoms of a UTI, such as burning during urination, frequent urination, cloudy or strong-smelling urine, pelvic pain, or fever.

Diabetes has a close relationship with urological health issues. People who have diabetes are more vulnerable to contracting urinary tract infections. They are also susceptible to bladder issues and sexual dysfunction. Diabetes is a debilitating condition that can worsen urologic problems because it affects blood flow and hampers the body's sensory functions.

Psoriasis is an antibiotic found naturally in the body that helps shield against UTIs. UTIs are more common in people with diabetes. High blood glucose levels caused by diabetes can lead to a deficiency of psoriasis.

Increasing Water Intake in Kidney Dialysis Patients

Drinking plenty of water and staying hydrated is necessary for kidney patients, as it allows the body to remove bacteria and toxins naturally. In this way, water intake can prevent illness.

Drinking water during and after an infection helps flush out the system and prevents future infections. It also helps remove bacteria that might otherwise reach the bladder and cause infection.

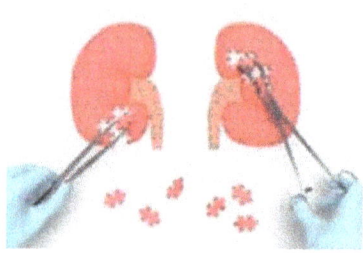

Filtration of hemodialysis fluids is also essential. This effectively eliminates bacteria and prevents endotoxin contamination. Using oxidants, especially chlorine or peracetic acid, is the most suitable method for removing bacteria and endotoxins in dialysis. Other effective methods include the use of ozone and heat sanitization, both of which are FDA-approved for dialysis applications.

Since people with diabetes are more vulnerable to urinary tract infections and bladder or sexual dysfunction, it is essential to exercise caution. Diabetes worsens urologic conditions because it affects the body's blood flow and sensory function. UTIs are not only more common in people with diabetes but also more severe, potentially causing renal abscesses, emphysematous cystitis, and renal papillary necrosis.

Uncovering the Root Causes of Dialysis Needs

Impact of Diabetes on the Immune System

For those with type 1 diabetes, the pancreas may stop producing insulin, which is required to regulate blood glucose levels. For people with type 2 diabetes, their cells become less sensitive to insulin.

In both conditions, excessive glucose levels can accumulate in the blood, negatively affecting the immune system. As mentioned earlier, high glucose levels reduce the amount of the natural antibiotic psoriasis, which serves as a shield against infection.

Urinary tract infections pose a greater risk in patients with type 2 diabetes mellitus. Resistant pathogens, immune impairments, and poor metabolic control increase the risk of UTIs in these patients.

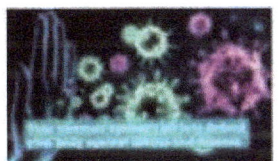

Infection Dangers for Chronic Stable Dialysis Patients

Dialysis patients face many dangers, including the risk of exposure to Staphylococcus aureus. This exposure can occur in dialysis centers, hospitals, or even rest homes.

The underlying issue is that the vascular access required during hemodialysis becomes a potential entry point for S. aureus. This risk is especially high when a central venous catheter is used, increasing the likelihood of sepsis compared to an arteriovenous fistula.

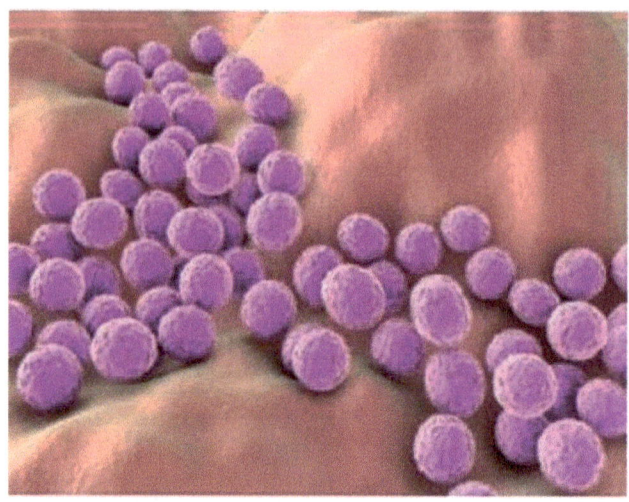

Activating the immune system's response

Staphylococcus aureus can infect the bloodstream, posing serious risks for hemodialysis patients. The human body's immune system responds by activating both the innate and adaptive immune systems.

The innate immune response is the body's first line of defense, acting rapidly and activating pathways that detect nonspecific microbial markers. Neutrophils, a type of white blood cell, are part of the body's nonspecific defense and play a crucial role in acute immune reactions. They are also a vital source of defense against S. aureus.

Uncovering the Root Causes of Dialysis Needs

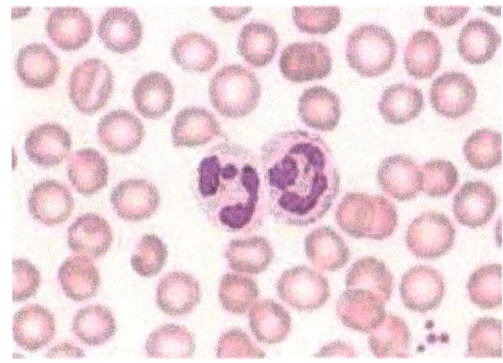

Neutrophils are white blood cells recognized for their role in chemotaxis. They form the human body's second line of nonspecific defense. As part of the immune system, they play an essential role in acute reactions and are a vital defense against *Staphylococcus aureus*.

It may surprise you, but 1 in 5 people are persistently colonized with *Staphylococcus aureus* bacteria. This is one of the leading causes of skin infections and a major reason for hospital-acquired infections, including the antibiotic-resistant strain MRSA.

Staphylococcus epidermidis is a member of the coagulase-negative Staphylococci group. It is recognized as a critical commensal organism on human skin and mucous membranes. Research has shown that it contributes to human health by fighting harmful microorganisms, offering benefits to the body.

Patients who require dialysis often have weakened immune systems. This makes it difficult for them to fight off infections. Despite this challenge, kidney patients cannot afford to skip their regularly scheduled dialysis treatments. Therefore, it is mandatory that they adhere completely to the precautions recommended by healthcare professionals.

The Importance of Mucus and Phlegm in the Human Body

Medically, mucus has one name, but in daily conversation, it is referred to by different terms. It could be called snot, the sticky goo that comes out of the nose during a cold, or phlegm, the thick mucus that clogs the lungs and causes coughing.

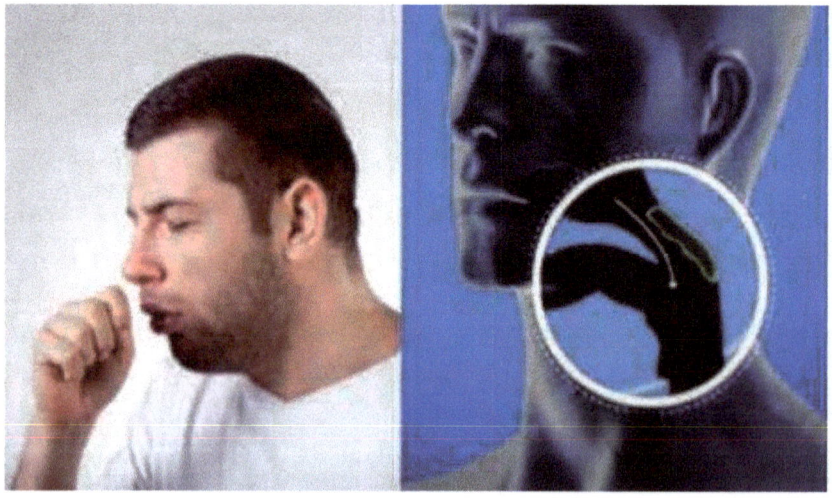

Mucus plays a vital role in the human body. Found in the respiratory tract, it warms and moistens inhaled air. It also ensures that mucus membrane cells and tiny hairs remain lubricated. Mucus acts as a

Uncovering the Root Causes of Dialysis Needs

barrier that defends the body by trapping pathogens, including infectious microorganisms and irritant particles, preventing them from entering the lungs.

The mucous membranes produce phlegm, which runs from the nose to the lungs. It helps trap viruses, allergens, and dust inhaled during breathing. These trapped particles are expelled from the body during exhalation. However, sometimes the body produces excess mucus, which leads to frequent coughing to clear the throat.

Does the color of the phlegm signify infection?

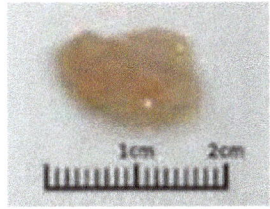

The color change depends on the severity and duration of the illness. If the phlegm is yellow or green, it may indicate that the body is fighting an infection. The color comes from white blood cells. Typically, phlegm starts yellow and may turn green as the infection progresses.

Ways to Treat Excess Mucus and Phlegm Buildup

Heating and drying out the nasal and respiratory passageways can help overcome this problem. Such treatments are often adopted in nursing homes. Another option is to manage the limited fluid intake

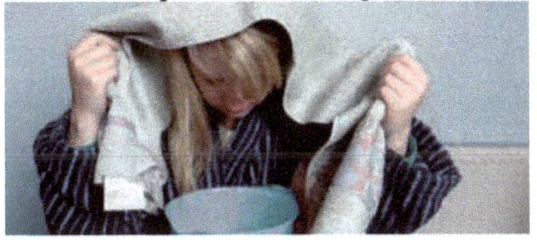

required by dialysis patients.

It is essential to keep the body hydrated to ensure mucus remains thin. If an individual falls sick, increasing fluid intake helps thin the mucus and drains the sinuses.

An easy solution is spending time in a steam-filled bathroom, which loosens and clears mucus from the nose and throat. Splashing hot water on the face also provides relief from sinus pressure.

Relief can also be obtained by applying a warm, wet washcloth. Heat plays a critical role in alleviating pain and pressure and can ease pounding sinus headaches. Inhaling steam with a damp cloth is another effective way to moisturize the nose and throat.

Boosting Immune Support for Dialysis Patients Through Medicinal and Nutritional Supplements

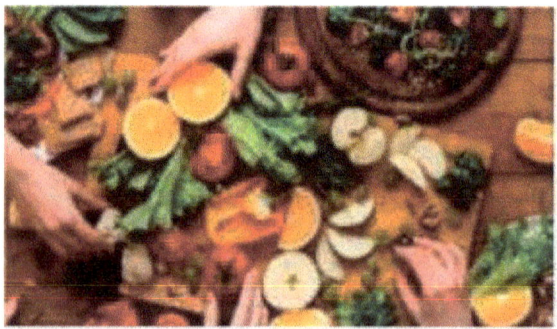

Patients requiring dialysis are at increased risk of infections. The risk of invasion by pathogens is high because they undergo hemodialysis frequently, which involves using catheters and sometimes needle insertions to access the bloodstream.

Supplements Dialysis Patients Need

Kidney patients require a high intake of certain water-soluble vitamins. This is why renal vitamins, which contain vitamins B1, B2, B6, B12, niacin, folic acid, biotin, a small dose of vitamin C, and pantothenic acid, are necessary to provide these nutrients.

Ways for Dialysis Patients to Improve Immunity

Different nutritional sources help boost the immune system and are essential for kidney health. Leafy greens such as spinach and kale are important sources of nutrients. Omega-3 fatty acids are also vital fats that support cell function.

Other powerful sources of vitamins include blueberries and strawberries. Patients with chronic kidney disease who require dialysis must avoid herbal remedies and over-the-counter supplements, as these can cause undesirable interactions with prescription medications.

Role of Seaweeds and Algae in Supporting the Immune System of Dialysis Patients

Seaweeds and microalgae contain pharmacologically active compounds such as phlorotannins, peptides, terpenes, fatty acids, and polysaccharides. These substances help fight bacterial invasion and support the immune system.

Seaweed is involved in the production of metabolites that help fight various environmental stressors. These compounds demonstrate several properties beneficial to the human body, including antiviral, antibacterial, antiprotozoal, and antifungal effects.

Tips on Boosting the Immune Systems of Dialysis Patients

Consume a diet rich in vitamin A, which is kidney-friendly. Examples include carrots, broccoli, eggs, and red bell peppers. An adequate intake of vitamin C is also recommended, with sources such as melons, berries, bell peppers, and citrus fruits. Vitamin E is essential and can be found in seeds, nuts, cereals, and peanut butter.

Many options are available to maintain a protein-rich diet. These include beef, chicken, beans, eggs, lamb, fish, turkey, veal, and lentils. Opting for natural, fresh meat is highly recommended, although frozen or canned meat can also be good options.

Sepsis in Brief: Symptoms, Entry Points, Potential Damage, and the Need to Control

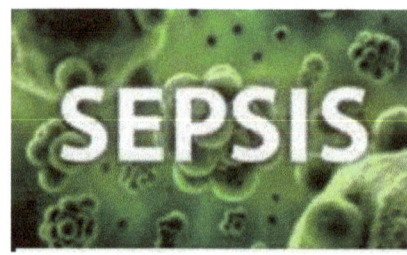

Sepsis refers to the body's extreme response to an infection. It occurs when an existing infection triggers a chain reaction throughout the body. Most infections that lead to sepsis start in organs such as the lungs, skin, or urinary tract. Sepsis is a severe, life-threatening condition that

Uncovering the Root Causes of Dialysis Needs

requires urgent medical attention.

Symptoms

Here are some of the symptoms of sepsis:

- Breathlessness
- Loss of consciousness
- A high or low body temperature
- Confusion or disorientation
- Slurred speech
- Cold and pale skin
- Heavy heartbeat
- Fast breathing

Sepsis may also lead to tissue damage, organ failure, and death. Healthcare professionals emphasize the importance of implementing safety protocols to keep the infection in check. These measures include assessing the sites accessed during hemodialysis through X-rays.

Response of the Immune System to Sepsis and Inflammation

The human body's immune system works to restrict an infection to one place, known as a localized infection. This is achieved by white blood cells produced by the body. White blood cells respond to an infection by traveling to the site to eliminate the germs responsible.

This process allows the body to fight the infection and prevent its spread.

However, this response also leads to tissue swelling, which is referred to as inflammation.

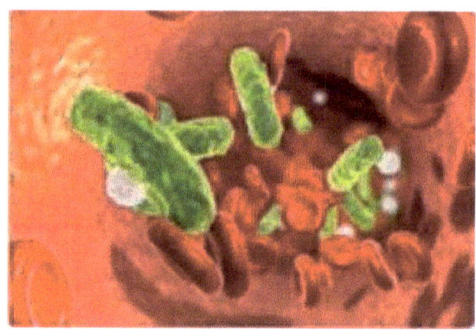

The infection may spread to other parts of the body if the immune system is weak. In cases of widespread inflammation, the tissue is at risk of damage, which may interfere with blood flow throughout the body. If blood flow is interrupted, it can cause blood pressure to drop to dangerously low levels and prevent oxygen from reaching all the organs and tissues. This situation may also occur if the infection is severe.

Sources of Infection (Entry Points)

Although sepsis may be triggered by an infection anywhere in the body, some common sites such as the lungs, abdomen, pelvis, and urinary tract are more likely to lead to sepsis.

Uncovering the Root Causes of Dialysis Needs

Spread of Sepsis by Extensive Use of AVF and CVC

There are three common vascular accesses for hemodialysis:

- Autologous arteriovenous fistulas (AVFs)
- Prosthetic grafts (AVGs)
- Central venous catheters (CVCs)

Of these three, professionals highly recommend AVF as the vascular access for hemodialysis because it is associated with lower morbidity and mortality rates compared to the other two options. Extensive use of AVF carries the least risk of spreading sepsis.

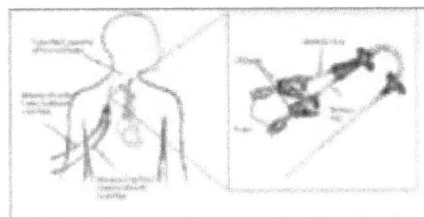

Starting dialysis via a CVC does not directly increase the risk of death. However, patients dialyzing through a catheter are more likely to die compared to those using an AVF. In contrast, fistulas have a lower risk of infection when compared to CVCs.

To avoid fistula malfunction and ensure high patency, AVFs have the potential to last longer than catheters. They are also associated with shorter hospital stays when patients are admitted for complications related to vascular access.

4: Managing the Essentials of Dialysis Treatment

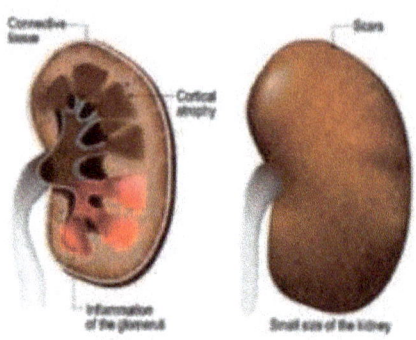

You probably don't think about your kidneys much, until something goes wrong. But deep inside your body, these quiet organs are hard at work, filtering out waste and keeping everything in balance. Now imagine what happens when that system starts to break down. That's where a condition like *glomerulonephritis* (GN) comes in, a word that sounds complicated but carries serious consequences.

Glomerulonephritis is a disease that inflames the tiny filters in your kidneys, known as *glomeruli*. These microscopic blood vessels do the heavy lifting of cleaning your blood and producing urine. When they're damaged, your whole system feels it. The inflammation can creep in suddenly (acute) or build up over time (chronic), sometimes with little warning. And if it goes untreated, the result can be devastating, kidney failure.

Uncovering the Root Causes of Dialysis Needs

The causes? They vary. GN might show up on its own, or it might tag along with other illnesses like lupus or diabetes. Sometimes it's triggered by infections, autoimmune disorders, or even lifestyle choices. Yes, what you eat and what you put in your body matters. Processed foods with artificial additives, preservatives like MSG or sodium nitrates, and excessive sugar or artificial sweeteners can contribute. Smoking, drug use (including marijuana and heroin), and even long-term nicotine exposure can also play a role.

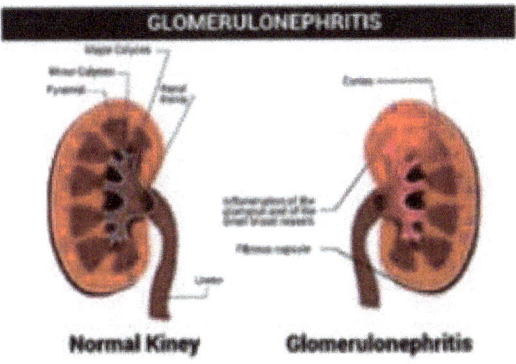

Some people experience mild cases that resolve on their own. But others aren't so lucky. The damage can be long-lasting, even permanent. That's why recognizing the signs early is so important.

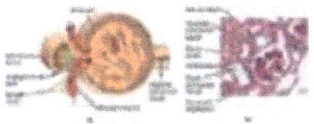

Let's take a step back and understand what glomeruli do. These tiny blood vessels are essential for filtering your blood and maintaining fluid balance. They help your body decide what to keep and what to flush out. When they're healthy, everything runs smoothly. But when inflammation sets in, waste starts to build up, and that's when trouble begins.

How Is Glomerulonephritis Classified?

There are two main types:

- **Acute Glomerulonephritis**, which shows up suddenly, sometimes after an infection like strep throat.
- **Chronic Glomerulonephritis**, which develops slowly and can silently damage your kidneys over the years.

Sometimes, an acute flare-up may resolve, only to return later in life as a chronic condition.

What Causes It?

Doctors don't always have clear answers. But here are some of the known or suspected triggers:

- **Genetics** – In rare cases, it runs in families.
- **Autoimmune diseases** – Conditions like lupus or anti-GBM disease can attack the kidneys.
- **Infections** – Hepatitis B or C, HIV, or bacterial infections such as endocarditis (affecting the heart valves).

- **Inflammatory disorders** – Certain diseases that inflame blood vessels can impact kidney function.

It's a complex picture, and that's what makes it so dangerous.

Signs and Symptoms to Watch For

The frustrating part? You might not feel anything at first. GN can be sneaky. But if your body *is* trying to tell you something, listen closely.

Here are some common red flags:

- Blood in the urine (which may look pink, red, or brown)
- Foamy urine (a sign of excess protein)
- Swelling in your face, hands, or legs
- High blood pressure
- Feeling tired, nauseous, or breaking out in a rash
- Trouble breathing
- Pain in your joints or abdomen
- Changes in how often you urinate, more or less than usual

If even one of these symptoms shows up, it's worth checking in with a doctor. Early detection could make all the difference.

Diagnosing Glomerulonephritis

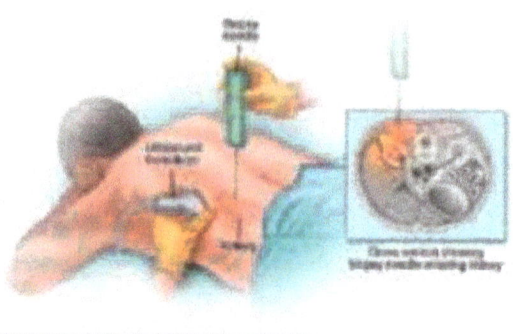

Like many kidney conditions, glomerulonephritis can be sneaky. The first signs of trouble often appear in subtle or unexpected ways, or sometimes not at all. That's part of what makes this disease so dangerous: it can silently damage the kidneys without producing obvious symptoms until it's progressed significantly.

When symptoms *do* occur, they may include:

- **Protein or blood in the urine** (often discovered through routine testing)
- **Foamy urine** (due to excess protein)
- **Swelling** in the face, hands, feet, or abdomen (caused by fluid retention)
- **High blood pressure**
- **Fatigue** or general malaise

Because these signs can be easy to miss or misattribute to other conditions, **early and accurate testing is essential**. A simple **urinalysis** can detect abnormal levels of protein or red blood cells, while **blood tests** can help assess kidney function by measuring levels of creatinine and blood urea nitrogen (BUN). These tests offer valuable insights into how well the kidneys are filtering waste from the blood.

In more complex or ambiguous cases, however, lab tests may not tell the full story. That's when a **kidney biopsy** becomes necessary. This procedure involves using a thin needle to extract a small sample of kidney tissue, which is then examined under a microscope. Though it may sound intimidating, the procedure is generally safe and minimally invasive. It allows doctors to:

- Identify the specific type of glomerulonephritis
- Determine the severity and stage of kidney damage
- Rule out other possible causes
- Guide the most effective treatment strategy

Ultimately, the goal of early diagnosis is to **preserve kidney function** and **prevent long-term complications**, including chronic kidney disease or kidney failure. If you or someone you love is experiencing unusual symptoms, or has risk factors such as diabetes, autoimmune disease, or a family history of kidney disorders, it's wise to consult a healthcare provider for screening.

Can You Prevent Glomerulonephritis?

Prevention isn't simple, mostly because we still don't fully understand what causes glomerulonephritis in all cases. But there *are* ways to reduce your risk.

It begins with basic but powerful steps:

- **Practice good hygiene.**
- **Have safe sex. Avoid unprotected intercourse and intravenous drug use.**
- **Avoid exposure to infections like hepatitis and HIV**, which are known to trigger GN.

If you're already living with chronic glomerulonephritis, you'll need to go even further. Managing blood pressure is critical. Adjusting your diet, especially by limiting protein, can help slow kidney damage.

Working with a renal dietitian can make all the difference. They'll guide you on what to eat, what to avoid, and how to nourish your body without overloading your kidneys.

Here are some practical steps to protect your health:

- Choose healthy, unprocessed foods
- Control blood pressure with a low-sodium diet, regular exercise, and medication

Uncovering the Root Causes of Dialysis Needs

- Prevent infections through careful hygiene
- Avoid needles for drugs or tattoos
- See a doctor for any suspicious infections, especially things like strep throat

Treatment Options for Glomerulonephritis

Sometimes, acute glomerulonephritis fades away on its own. In mild cases, temporary care might be enough. But if things worsen, more aggressive treatment may be needed.

For example, if fluid builds up dangerously, doctors might use an artificial kidney machine (dialysis) to remove it. This helps stabilize blood pressure and prevents kidney failure.

One important note: antibiotics can treat infections, but they can't cure glomerulonephritis itself, unless the root cause is a bacterial infection.

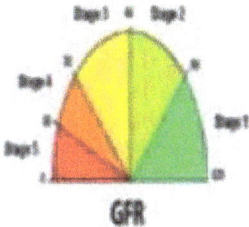

When the illness progresses rapidly, stronger interventions are required. Doctors may use high doses of immunosuppressive medications to slow the immune system. They might also use plasmapheresis, a special blood-filtering process that removes harmful proteins from the bloodstream.

Living With Chronic Glomerulonephritis

Chronic GN doesn't have a one-size-fits-all cure. But there are steps you can take to protect what kidney function you have left.

Doctors often recommend:

- **Reducing protein, salt, and potassium intake**
- **Managing blood pressure** vigilantly
- **Treating swelling** with diuretics (also called water pills)
- **Taking calcium supplements**, when needed
- **Avoiding drug abuse**, especially anything involving needles
- **Staying away from foods packed with artificial additives and preservatives**

Be mindful of what goes into your body. Read the labels. Avoid sodium nitrites, artificial colors, high fructose corn syrup, and chemical sweeteners. Instead, reach for foods preserved with natural ingredients, like garlic, vinegar, or citrus extracts.

Uncovering the Root Causes of Dialysis Needs

Medications That May Help

Doctors may also prescribe medicines to help manage your condition, reduce complications, and improve your quality of life. These include:

- **ACE inhibitors** (angiotensin-converting enzyme inhibitors)
- **ARBs** (angiotensin II receptor blockers)
- **Calcium channel blockers**
- **Diuretics**
- **Alpha-adrenergic agonists**
- **Beta-adrenergic blockers**

Each has a purpose, some lower blood pressure, others reduce swelling or protect your heart. The goal is always the same: slow the disease, protect the kidneys, and give you the best chance at a full

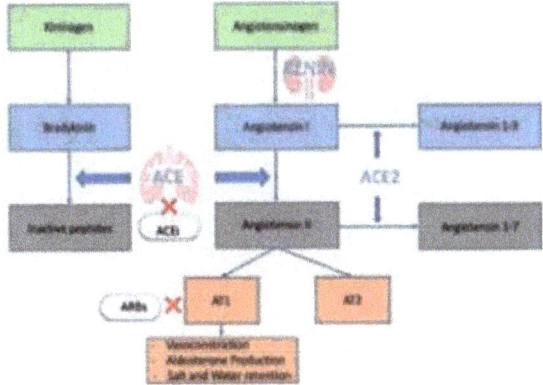

and healthy life.

Complications of Glomerulonephritis

When glomerulonephritis strikes, it doesn't just affect the kidneys, it disrupts the body's entire internal balance.

The disease attacks the nephrons, those tiny but vital filters within the kidneys. Once damaged, they can no longer properly remove waste or toxins from the bloodstream. The result? Harmful substances build up. Vital proteins and red blood cells are lost in urine. Essential nutrients and minerals fall out of balance.

It's not just a kidney problem. It becomes a full-body crisis.

The Hidden Dangers: Complications of Glomerulonephritis

One of the most alarming consequences is **acute kidney failure**, a sudden, rapid decline in kidney function. This often occurs when glomerulonephritis is triggered by an infection.

In this critical state, the body can no longer eliminate excess fluids or toxins. The waste floods the system. If left untreated, it can lead to death.

Dialysis is required immediately to take over the kidneys' job. But there's a silver lining: with timely intervention, kidney function can return.

Another serious outcome is chronic kidney disease. This happens when inflammation persists over time, slowly but steadily eroding

Uncovering the Root Causes of Dialysis Needs

kidney function. If the damage continues, the disease can progress to end-stage renal disease, where survival depends on dialysis or a kidney transplant.

The Chain Reaction: High Blood Pressure and Nephrotic Syndrome

When glomeruli are damaged, blood pressure often rises. Inflammation disturbs the filtering mechanism, creating pressure in the blood vessels. Over time, this pressure only worsens the condition.

In other cases, glomerulonephritis can trigger nephrotic syndrome. This is when large amounts of protein leak into the urine, leaving too little in the bloodstream. That protein is essential, it helps regulate cholesterol and fluid balance. Its absence causes swelling in the hands, feet, face, and abdomen.

Worse still, nephrotic syndrome can increase cholesterol, raise blood pressure, and, though rare, lead to blood clots in the kidney's vessels.

Nourishing the Body: Diet for Acute Glomerulonephritis

Food can become medicine when chosen wisely. For those dealing with acute glomerulonephritis, the right diet supports recovery.

Recommended Foods:

- **Lean proteins**: fish, poultry

Dialysis Champions

- **Legumes**: chickpeas, soybeans
- **Nuts**: peanuts (in moderation)
- **Fruits**: apples, watermelon, bananas, oranges, pears
- **Vegetables**: tomatoes, potatoes, lettuce
- **Grains**: rice, whole-grain cereals
- **Snacks**: low-salt options
- **Preservation**: avoid chemical preservatives; opt for natural methods like freezing, heating, or moisture control

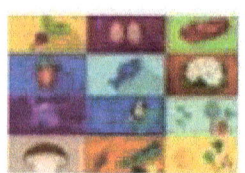

A **low-sodium diet** is essential to reduce strain on the kidneys.

The Hidden Link: Drug Abuse and Kidney Damage

The link between illicit drug use and glomerulonephritis is undeniable, and deeply concerning.

Many renal disorders are rooted in substance abuse. Among intravenous drug users, post-infectious glomerulonephritis and hepatitis-related glomerulonephritis are tragically common.

Uncovering the Root Causes of Dialysis Needs

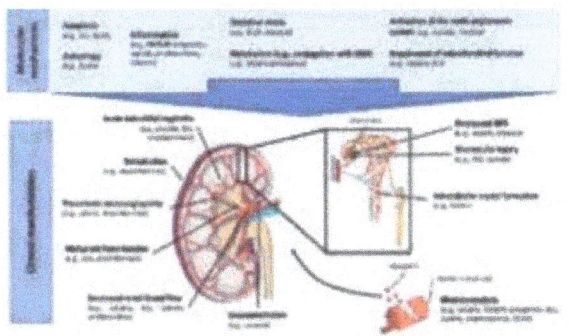

Drugs can provoke inflammation in the glomeruli, the renal tubules, and the surrounding tissues. Over time, this inflammation leads to renal scarring and fibrosis, permanent damage that silently destroys kidney function.

Uremic Toxins: The Invisible Threat

Your kidneys are remarkable, they filter the waste your body doesn't need. But when they fail, the waste doesn't leave. It stays.

And it poisons you.

These uremic toxins come from your body's natural metabolic processes. A healthy kidney eliminates them, keeping levels in blood and tissue low. But when kidney function drops, these toxins accumulate. The result is uremia, a toxic state often seen in patients with chronic or end-stage kidney disease.

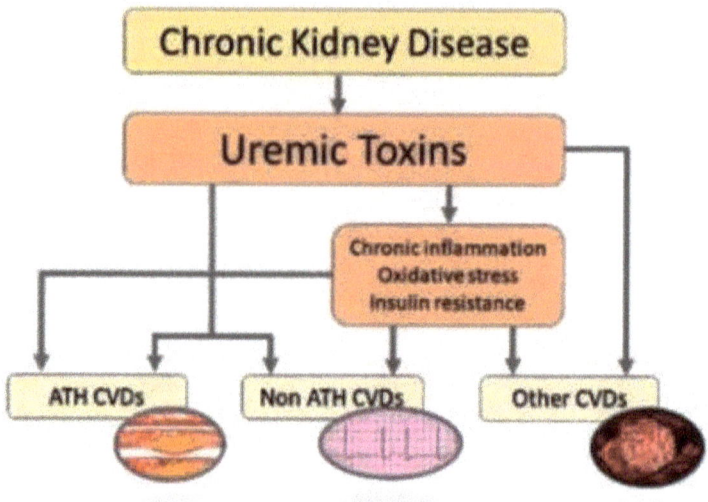

What Are Uremic Toxins?

They fall into three categories:

1. **Small solutes**
2. **Middle molecules**
3. **Protein-bound toxins**

These toxins, organic or inorganic, build up in patients with impaired kidney function. Together, they lead to uremic syndrome, a condition that affects nearly every organ system.

Uremic toxins are shaped by what you eat. They're heavily influenced by:

- **Protein intake** (animal and plant-based)

Uncovering the Root Causes of Dialysis Needs

- **Gut microbiota**
- **Enterohepatic circulation**

Research shows that small and middle molecules are usually removed via glomerular filtration, while protein-bound toxins require tubular secretion.

But when the kidneys are weak, these systems fail. And the toxins stay.

Dialysis has long been a lifeline, an essential tool in removing low-molecular-weight uremic toxins from the body. But its strength ends there.

Protein-bound uremic toxins, the larger and more dangerous kind, often remain behind. The standard dialysis membranes simply can't filter them out. And so, they linger, silently damaging the body, organ by organ.

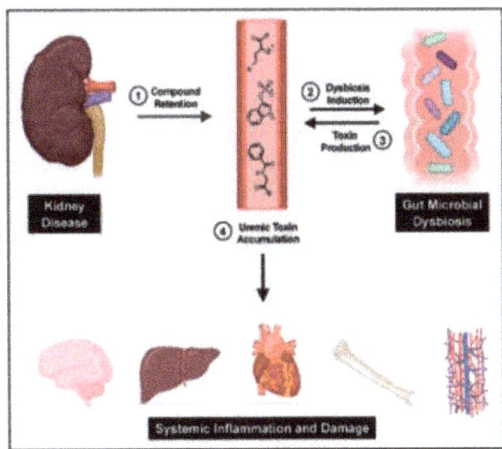

A Growing Awareness: Medical Interest in Uremic Syndrome

Over the past two decades, a shift has occurred in the medical community. Doctors, researchers, and nephrologists have begun to pay closer attention to uremic syndrome and its long-term impact on patients with chronic kidney disease (CKD).

But the truth is unsettling.

Despite extensive research, the full nature of uremic toxins remains elusive. What we do know is this: these organic residual compounds, once trapped in the body, begin to circulate through the bloodstream. From there, they infiltrate vital organs, especially the kidneys and heart, wreaking havoc.

As chronic kidney disease progresses, these toxins accumulate. And with them come irreversible functional changes throughout the body.

Why Protein-Bound Toxins Matter

Unlike smaller molecules, protein-bound toxins are especially hard to eliminate. Dialysis, the very process designed to cleanse the blood, cannot reach them. The membranes used simply aren't equipped to break the bonds that hold these toxins tight.

This is why researchers have turned to alternatives, newer technologies and advanced dialysis methods, in search of a better solution.

Uncovering the Root Causes of Dialysis Needs

New Frontiers: High-Flux and MCO Dialysis

Among the promising innovations is high-flux dialysis. This method uses specially designed membranes to remove medium-sized molecules, improving clearance beyond traditional dialysis.

Still, there's a limit.

For molecules larger than 15 kilodaltons (kDa), such as myoglobin (17 kDa) and FGF-23 (32 kDa), even high-flux dialysis falls short.

That's where Medium Cut-Off (MCO) membranes come in.

Recent studies comparing high-flux hemodialysis to MCO membrane hemodialysis revealed something striking: patients using MCO dialyzers had significantly lower levels of myoglobin and β2-microglobulin after just a few sessions. In other words, MCO dialysis works, and it works better.

However, there's a catch. Some studies noted that MCO dialysis may reduce serum albumin levels over time. The long-term significance of this drop is still unclear, and further investigation is needed.

Uremic Toxins and the Mind: Altered Mental Status

Chronic kidney disease doesn't just attack the body, it invades the mind.

Patients often suffer from a range of neuropsychiatric disorders: Depression. Anxiety. Cognitive decline.

These aren't just side effects. They're deeply woven into the experience of living with CKD, impacting mental well-being and eroding quality of life. And sadly, they come with a heavy toll, increased hospitalization rates and higher mortality.

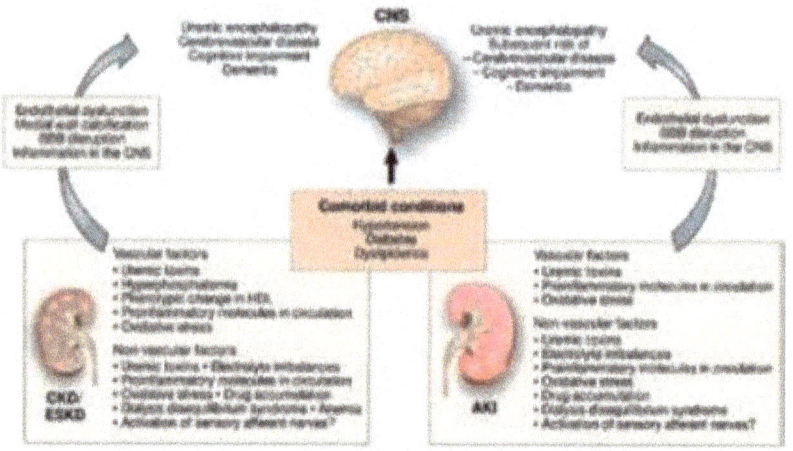

But what's behind it?

Emerging evidence points to a common culprit: uremic toxins. Accumulating in the bloodstream, they appear to trigger a cascade of neurological changes, particularly in regions affected by cerebrovascular disease.

Curiously, studies show no strong link between cognitive decline and traditional vascular risk factors like diabetes and hypertension in CKD patients. This suggests a distinct, underlying pathology, one that may connect renal disease and brain dysfunction at a deeper level.

Uncovering the Root Causes of Dialysis Needs

Even children with CKD show signs of neuropsychiatric complications, proving the link isn't just about age or comorbidities. It's a direct and devastating result of uremia.

The Evidence is Clear: Cognitive Decline and Kidney Function

The numbers speak volumes.

For every 15 ml/min/1.73 m² decrease in glomerular filtration rate (GFR), there's a cognitive decline equivalent to aging three years.

It's not just a statistic, it's a warning. CKD is not merely a physical disease. It is a neurological risk factor, silently stealing years of mental clarity and emotional stability.

Psychiatric Disorders: An Overlooked Crisis

CKD patients are three times more likely to be hospitalized for psychiatric conditions, **depression, anxiety, substance use disorders**, than those with other chronic illnesses.

And the impact is cruelly cyclical.

Uremic toxins cause cognitive and emotional distress. That distress leads to reduced self-care, increased isolation, and worsening health. The mind suffers as much as the body, and both spiral together.

Uremic toxins do more than harm the kidneys, they reach the brain, inflicting damage that surpasses the effects of hemodynamic shifts or lipid metabolism disturbances. As kidney function declines, these toxins accumulate, triggering a cascade of consequences: systemic inflammation, cardiac failure, anemia, anorexia, immune dysfunction, and perhaps most tragically, neurological and cognitive decline.

One of the most haunting aspects of uremic toxicity is its ability to breach the brain's last line of defense, the blood-brain barrier (BBB). Once across, it disrupts the fragile neurological balance, causing neurodegeneration and cognitive impairment. Among the chief culprits are para-cresyl sulfate (PCS), fibroblast growth factor 23 (FGF23), phosphate, and indoxyl sulfate (IS). These uremic toxins don't just harm, they attack the very system that governs who we are: our minds, our memories, our personalities. The brain's monoaminergic system, which plays a critical role in mood regulation, is especially vulnerable to these toxins.

p-Cresyl sulfate (PCS)   Indoxyl sulfate (IS)

But the damage doesn't stop with toxins.

Uncovering the Root Causes of Dialysis Needs

"Your CRP levels are elevated," the doctor said, eyebrows knitted with concern.

"What does that mean?" the patient asked, gripping the edge of the hospital bed.

"It means your body is inflamed, something is wrong. Possibly an infection, or even a chronic condition."

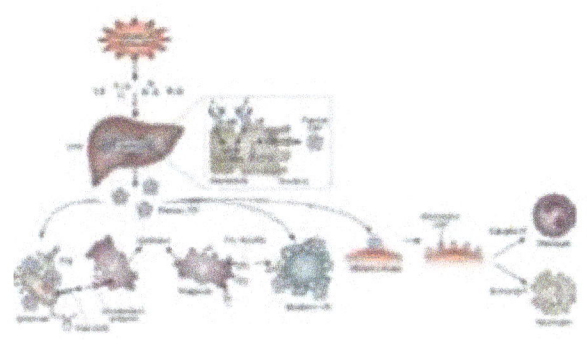

C-reactive protein (CRP) is a silent alarm bell, sounded by the liver in response to inflammation. In healthy individuals, CRP levels remain low. But when inflammation sets in, whether from infection, injury, or disease, the liver floods the bloodstream with CRP.

One of the more subtle yet sinister contributors to chronic inflammation is diet, specifically, a high-sugar diet. This kind of diet becomes a playground for opportunistic invaders: fungi, bacteria, and viruses. These pathogens latch onto sugars coating the surfaces of our cells, multiply, and inflame tissues. The liver responds by ramping up CRP, intensifying the inflammation and compounding the damage.

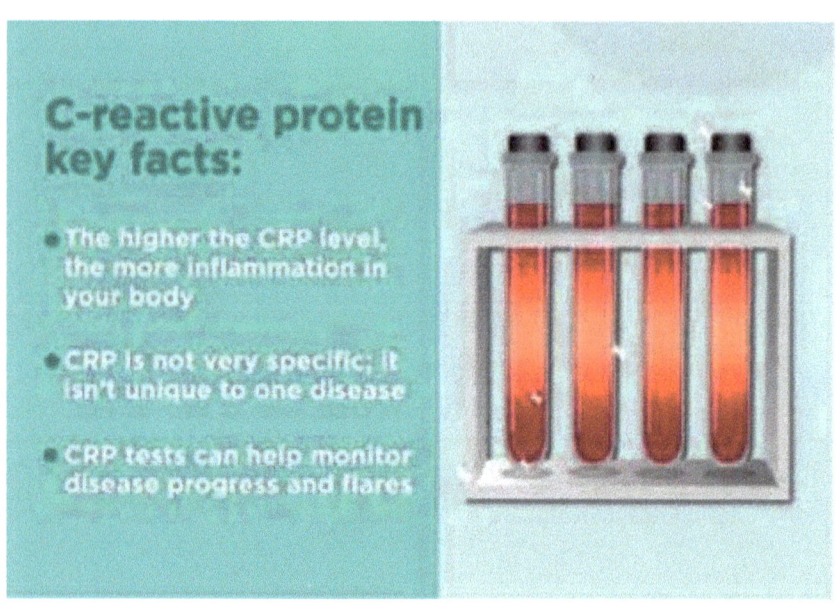

This dangerous cycle stems from a metabolic pathway called gluconeogenesis, the body's process of generating glucose from non-carbohydrate sources when dietary intake is insufficient. When hijacked by pathogens, this process floods the body with sugar, leading to hyperglycemia, an excessive amount of glucose in the blood. This isn't just a blood sugar issue, it's a full-blown systemic crisis.

Hyperglycemia alters mental status.

"I've been feeling foggy, confused. Sometimes I forget simple

things. Is it the diabetes?"

"Yes," the doctor replied gently. **"High blood sugar doesn't just affect your body, it affects your brain too."**

When blood sugar levels soar, patients with diabetes often report changes in mood, confusion, even episodes of delirium. This isn't anecdotal, it's documented. The brain's chemistry shifts, impairing attention, memory, and emotional regulation.

But the consequences of ignoring hyperglycemia can be even more devastating.

Without intervention, the body, starved of usable glucose, begins to break down fats to survive. This produces ketones, which, in high concentrations, acidify the blood, a dangerous condition known as diabetic ketoacidosis, or "diabetic coma." It can strike quickly and can be fatal.

The relationship between sugar, inflammation, and the mind is no longer speculation, it's science. Studies show a direct correlation between high sugar intake and increased levels of CRP. Interestingly, this relationship does **not** exist with the intake of fruits, vegetables, or even essential vitamins and minerals. It's sugar alone that feeds the fire.

Cytokines, small proteins involved in cell signaling, trigger the liver to produce CRP. When inflammation becomes chronic, CRP levels linger between 1.0 and 10.0 mg/dL, often observed in autoimmune diseases like lupus, rheumatoid arthritis, or systemic inflammation from chronic infections.

This is not just about blood sugar readings, it's about the way we live, eat, and care for ourselves. High glucose levels are now associated with increased deposits of **beta-amyloid** proteins in the brain, protein fragments known to cluster between nerve cells, impeding communication and contributing to the neurodegeneration seen in Alzheimer's disease.

Among the many conditions triggered by persistently high blood sugar, one of the lesser-known threats is *Rheumatoid Arthritis*, a chronic inflammatory disorder that can severely affect your joints and overall mobility.

The Silent Link: Hyperglycemia and Dementia

If you or someone you love is living with either hypoglycemia or hyperglycemia, there's a sobering fact you need to know: the risk of developing dementia is six times higher than for those with stable blood sugar levels.

Why? Because extreme fluctuations in blood glucose can take a toll on the brain. Studies have shown that older adults with type 1 diabetes are especially vulnerable. The damage from repeated glycemic episodes doesn't just affect the body, it silently erodes memory, cognitive function, and emotional balance.

Uncovering the Root Causes of Dialysis Needs

CRP Test: A Window Into Inflammation

When the body is fighting an infection or dealing with chronic disease, it often sends out a signal, in the form of *C-reactive protein* (CRP).

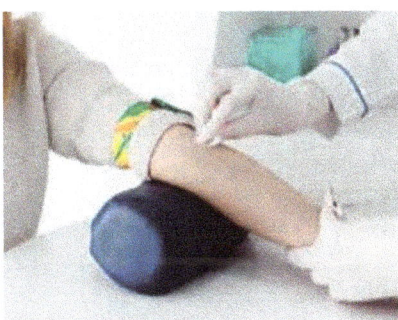

A CRP test can detect and monitor inflammation caused by both acute infections and long-term illnesses.

If you're experiencing symptoms like:

- Fever or chills
- A rapid heartbeat or quickened breath
- Nausea and vomiting

…it may indicate a bacterial infection, and a CRP test becomes essential.

But CRP isn't just for identifying what's wrong, it's also a powerful tool to measure progress. When CRP levels drop, it's a hopeful sign: treatment is working, or your body is beginning to heal. For those battling chronic inflammatory conditions, CRP tests help doctors track the disease and tailor future treatment plans.

Pectin: A Natural Ally for Blood Sugar, Fat, and Weight Management

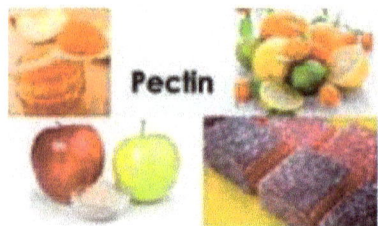

Found in everyday fruits like apples, pears, guavas, plums, and citrus, *pectin* is more than just dietary fiber, it's a silent healer.

This soluble fiber does three powerful things for your body:

1. Regulates Blood Sugar:

In studies involving mice, pectin lowered blood sugar and improved insulin sensitivity, crucial for managing type 2 diabetes.

2. Reduces Blood Fat:

Pectin binds to cholesterol in the digestive system, preventing its absorption. The result? Lower cholesterol levels and a reduced risk of heart disease.

3. Promotes Healthy Weight:

Pectin-rich foods are naturally filling and lower in calories. Increased fiber intake is directly linked to a reduced risk of obesity. Animal studies also show that pectin supplements help burn fat and support weight loss.

How to Add Pectin to Your Diet

Uncovering the Root Causes of Dialysis Needs

It's easy: eat more fresh fruits and vegetables. Apples are a great start.

But beware, commercial jams and jellies might *claim* to be high in pectin, but they're usually packed with sugar and contain only trace amounts of beneficial fiber. Stick to whole foods for the real benefits.

When Pathogens Thrive: The Role of Hypoxia in Infection

Here's a surprising twist: oxygen deprivation, *hypoxia*, can actually help certain infections grow stronger.

How? Bacterial and fungal pathogens thrive in low-oxygen environments. They use respiration to consume what little oxygen remains, weakening the immune system's natural defenses.

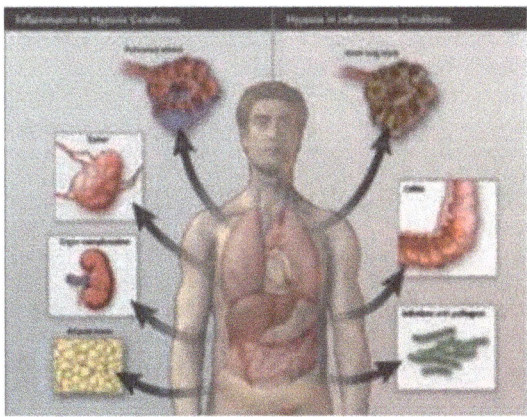

Macrophages and neutrophils, two key immune cells, rely on oxygen to generate reactive oxygen species (ROS), their main weapon against invaders. When hypoxia sets in, their effectiveness drops, and pathogens gain the upper hand.

Regarding immune modulatory effects, besides its antimicrobial activity, ROS is also a precursor to the progression of inflammatory diseases. This occurs due to the increased impact on biological structures and the promotion of pro-inflammatory cytokines.

Different infectious disease studies have concluded that pathogens stand to benefit from hypoxia. Aerobic pathogens refer to bacteria that find a way to grow and live in the presence of oxygen.

Since bacteria lack intracellular compartments (organelles), cellular respiration occurs in the cytoplasm and at the plasma membrane. Aerobic respiration utilizes oxygen in this process.

Some aerobic bacteria use aerobic respiration, including obligate aerobes, facultative aerobes, microaerophiles, and aerotolerant aerobes.

Either surgical drainage or debridement is used to treat aerobic infections. Antibiotics may also be used to treat certain infections caused by bacteria. However, some bacterial infections may be treated without the use of antibiotics.

Uncovering the Root Causes of Dialysis Needs

5: Inflammation and Pain

Inflammation: An Overview

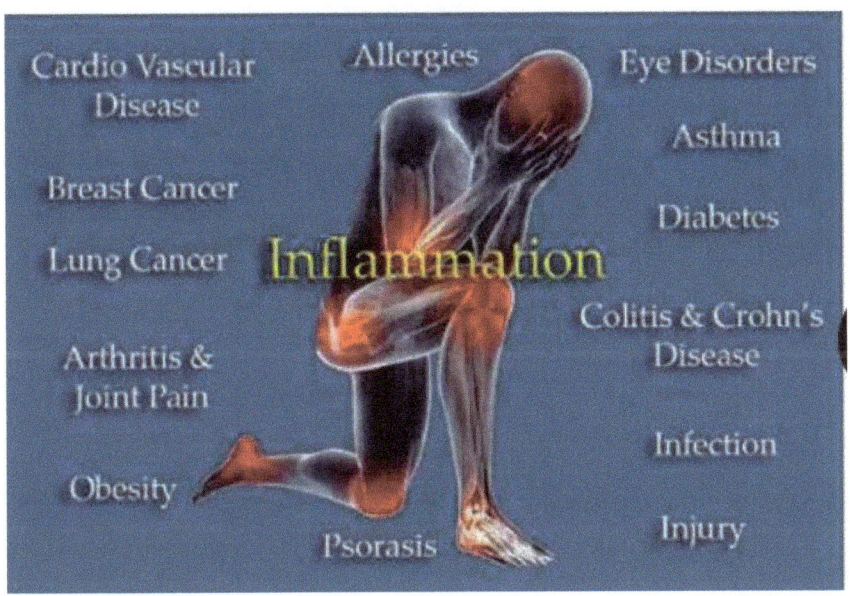

Inflammation is an essential part of the body's natural defense system. It plays a vital role in the healing process, protecting us from harm and restoring health after injury or infection.

When the body detects an injury or encounters an intruder, such as 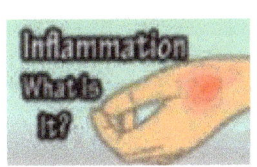 a thorn, an irritant, or a pathogen, it launches a biological response aimed at eliminating the threat. Pathogens can include viruses, bacteria, and other harmful organisms that invade the body and trigger infection.

How the Body Responds

The immune system sends its first responders: inflammatory cells and cytokines. These substances act quickly. Cytokines stimulate additional inflammatory cells, which then rush to the affected area, trapping harmful invaders and initiating the healing process.

This intricate response often leads to familiar symptoms, pain, redness, swelling, bruising, and heat, all signs that the body is fighting to heal.

When the Body Attacks Itself

Sometimes, however, this defense system turns inward. The body mistakenly identifies its own cells and tissues as threats, triggering an unnecessary immune response. This is the root of autoimmune diseases.

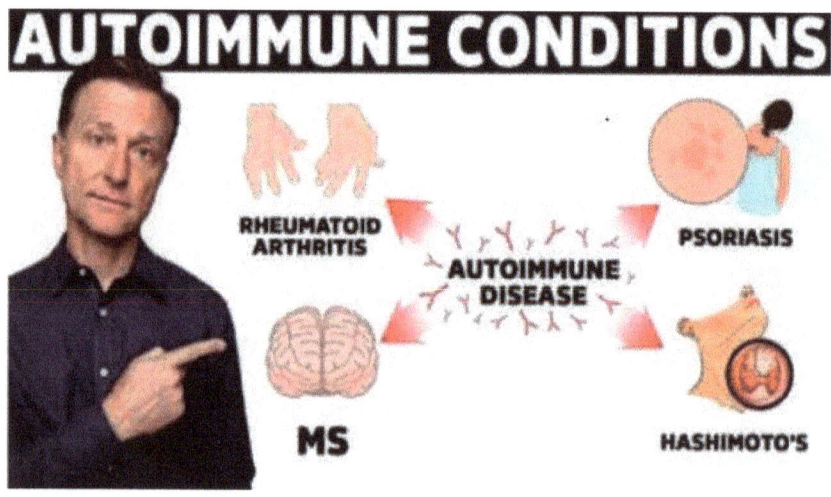

For instance, in type 1 diabetes, the immune system attacks insulin-producing cells in the pancreas. Experts also believe chronic inflammation plays a significant role in other long-term conditions, including type 2 diabetes, heart disease, obesity, and metabolic syndrome. In such cases, individuals often show elevated levels of inflammation markers in their blood.

Measuring Inflammation: The Role of Biomarkers

Inflammation can be measured through biomarkers, specific substances in the body that indicate the presence and intensity of an inflammatory response.

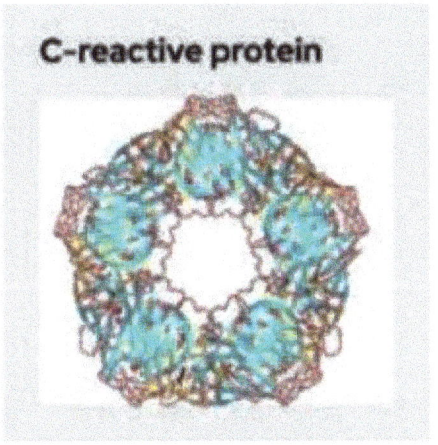

One of the most commonly used biomarkers is *C-reactive protein (CRP)*. When inflammation is present, CRP levels rise. This is why the CRP test is a critical tool for doctors in diagnosing and monitoring inflammation-related conditions.

It's worth noting that CRP levels tend to be higher in older adults and individuals with obesity or cancer. Diet and physical activity also influence these levels.

Types of Inflammation: Acute vs. Chronic

Inflammation is typically classified into two types: *acute* and *chronic*.

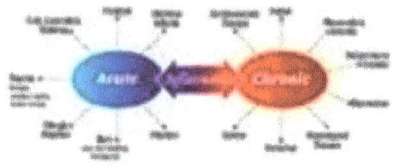

Acute Inflammation: The Immediate Response

Acute inflammation is the body's rapid response to injury or infection. It typically develops within hours or days and resolves in a short time. This type of inflammation is marked by five key signs:

- **Pain** – constant or triggered by touch
- **Redness** – due to increased blood flow to the area
- **Loss of function** – especially in joints or affected limbs
- **Swelling** – caused by fluid buildup (edema)
- **Heat** – as blood rushes to the injured tissue

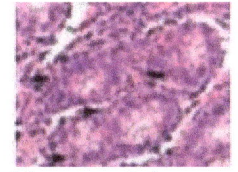 However, these signs are not always visible. Sometimes, inflammation is "silent." A person may feel unwell, fatigued, or develop a fever without noticing any external symptoms.

In some cases, symptoms may last longer than expected. This stage, called *subacute inflammation*, can extend from two to six weeks.

What Triggers Acute Inflammation?

When the body recognizes damage or an invading organism, it initiates a powerful defense. Plasma proteins accumulate at the site, causing swelling. White blood cells, particularly *neutrophils* (a type of *leukocyte*), move to the affected area. These cells are equipped with specialized molecules designed to fight off pathogens.

To support their access, the body widens tiny blood vessels, allowing more leukocytes and plasma proteins to reach the damaged tissue quickly.

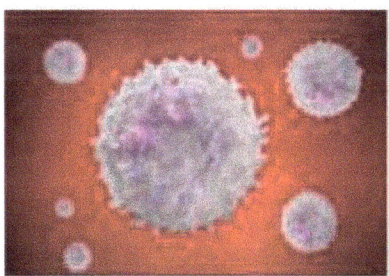

How long it takes for symptoms to appear depends on the cause, sometimes within hours, sometimes days. Common triggers of acute inflammation include:

- An ingrown toenail
- A sore throat
- Physical trauma
- Acute bronchitis
- A wound
- Appendicitis

Chronic Inflammation: When Healing Turns Harmful

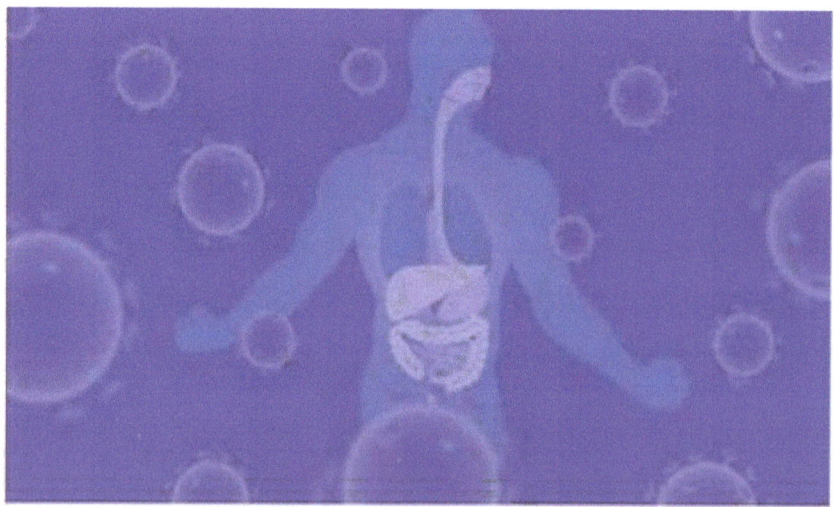

Unlike acute inflammation, which resolves quickly after an injury or infection, chronic inflammation lingers, sometimes for months, even years. This prolonged immune response is not just a symptom; it becomes a condition in itself, often linked to serious diseases such as:

- Allergies
- Arthritis and other joint diseases
- Cardiovascular conditions
- Psoriasis
- Diabetes
- Rheumatoid arthritis

The symptoms of chronic inflammation, persistent pain, fatigue, and discomfort, vary depending on the specific illness but share a common root: an immune system that doesn't know when to stop.

Why Does Chronic Inflammation Happen?

There isn't just one answer. Chronic inflammation can arise for many reasons:

- **Hypersensitivity:** For some, even harmless substances are perceived as threats. Allergies are a classic example, where the immune system overreacts to pollen, dust, or certain foods.

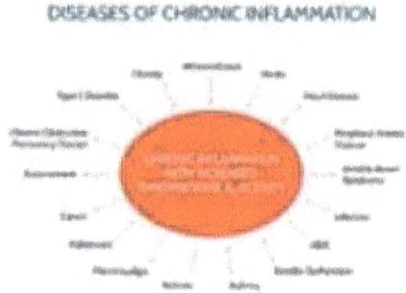

- **Prolonged exposure to irritants:** Constant contact with irritants, like industrial chemicals, can slowly damage tissues and spark lasting inflammation.

- **Autoimmunity:** Sometimes, the body mistakes its own healthy tissues for enemies. This misfire leads to autoimmune diseases, such as psoriasis or rheumatoid arthritis.

- **Genetic disorders:** In rare cases, inherited conditions, known as autoinflammatory diseases, disrupt immune function. Behçet's disease is one such example.

- **Unresolved acute inflammation:** When the body fails to fully recover from a short-term inflammatory response, the healing process remains incomplete, and chronic inflammation sets in.

Uncovering the Root Causes of Dialysis Needs

Nociceptors: The Body's Pain Detectors

Pain is one of inflammation's loudest messengers, and nociceptors are the sensory receptors responsible for detecting it. These tiny nerve endings respond to signals from damaged tissues and chemical changes in the body, relaying urgent messages to the brain.

What Are Nociceptors?

Nociceptors are free nerve endings found throughout the body, on the skin, in muscles, joints, and even bones. They act as sentinels, always on guard for signs of danger.

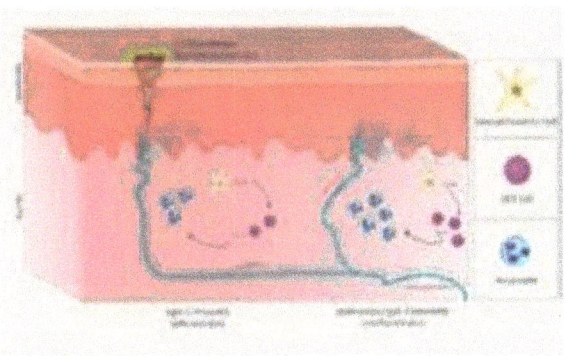

When damage occurs, these receptors activate and send electrical signals through the spinal cord to the brain. For example, if you stub your toe, nociceptors in the skin fire off a message that travels through peripheral nerves and reaches the brain in a split second. That's how you feel pain, fast and unmistakable.

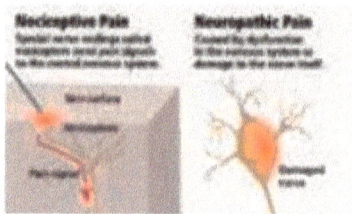

Types of Nociceptors

Nociceptors are categorized based on the type of stimulus they respond to:

- **Thermal Nociceptors**

    These detect extreme temperatures. Touching a hot stove or stepping onto ice can instantly trigger their response.

- **Mechanical Nociceptors**

    Activated by intense pressure or physical distortion, like pulling a hamstring or twisting an ankle. They respond when tissues are stretched beyond their capacity.

- **Chemical Nociceptors**

    These react to chemical irritants, whether from within (such as compounds released during tissue damage) or from external exposure (like bleach or chili oil).

- **Silent Nociceptors**

    Found mostly in internal organs, these remain inactive until inflammation occurs. Once triggered, they begin responding

Uncovering the Root Causes of Dialysis Needs

to chemical, thermal, or mechanical stimuli.

How Pain Travels: The Transmission Process

Beyond the type of stimulus, nociceptors are also classified by how quickly they transmit signals. This speed is determined by the kind of nerve fibers they contain, known as axons.

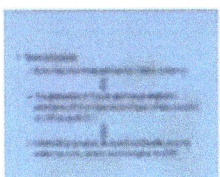

- **A Fibers (A-delta axons)**

    These fibers are coated in a protective sheath called *myelin*, which allows signals to travel quickly. They are responsible for the sharp, immediate pain you feel after a sudden injury.

- **C Fibers**

    Lacking a myelin sheath, these fibers transmit signals more slowly. They carry signals associated with lingering, burning pain.

The Two Phases of Pain

When you cut your finger or touch something hot, two different pain signals follow:

1. **Fast Pain (First Phase)**

    This sharp, pricking pain is carried by A fibers and felt

almost instantly. It's your body's urgent alarm, prompting a quick reaction, like pulling your hand away.

2. **Slow Pain (Second Phase)**

A few moments later, the deeper, burning pain sets in. This is the domain of C fibers. It persists long after the initial stimulus ends, reminding you that healing is still underway.

This delay explains why pain seems to intensify moments after an injury. The aching sensations in sore muscles or stomach cramps are also traced to the slower transmission of C fibers, especially those in internal organs.

The Role of Manuka Honey in Fighting Bacteria and Reducing Inflammation

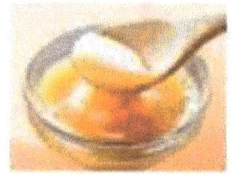

Manuka honey is produced by bees that pollinate the tea tree, scientifically known as *Leptospermum scoparium*, a plant native to Australia and New Zealand. What sets this honey apart is its unique combination of properties that offer notable health benefits, particularly in supporting wound healing and fighting infections.

Uncovering the Root Causes of Dialysis Needs

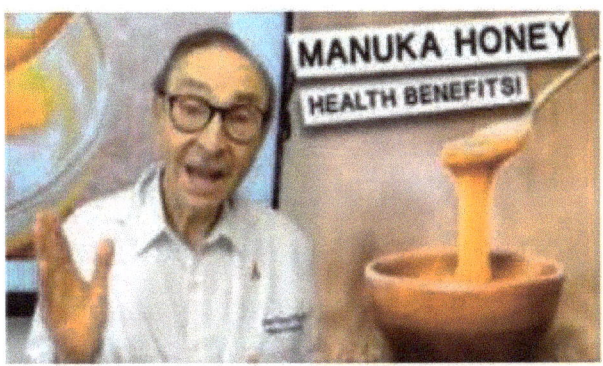

Rich in both antioxidant and antibiotic compounds, Manuka honey has been found effective in reducing inflammation and combating disease-causing bacteria. Its therapeutic value has made it a go-to remedy for conditions such as joint pain, inflamed arthritis, wounds, ulcers, and burns.

Honey has long been used across cultures as a natural remedy to prevent infection and promote healing. However, recent scientific interest in Manuka honey has highlighted its particularly potent antibacterial and anti-inflammatory effects. These properties have led to its incorporation into various wound dressings and its growing use as a dietary supplement for overall health.

Research suggests that Manuka honey can serve as a valuable biomaterial additive, showing promise in reducing acute inflammation and promoting tissue repair. While hydrogen peroxide accounts for the antibacterial effects of most honeys, Manuka honey offers something more.

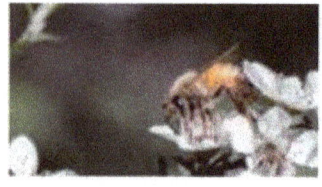 Its power lies in a compound called **methylglyoxal (MGO)**, which is formed from **dihydroxyacetone (DHA)**, a substance found in high concentrations in the nectar of Manuka flowers. This gives Manuka honey its unique antibacterial potency, enabling it to protect the body from bacterial damage, enhance tissue healing, and activate an anti-inflammatory response to ease pain and swelling.

Pus: A Natural Response to Infection

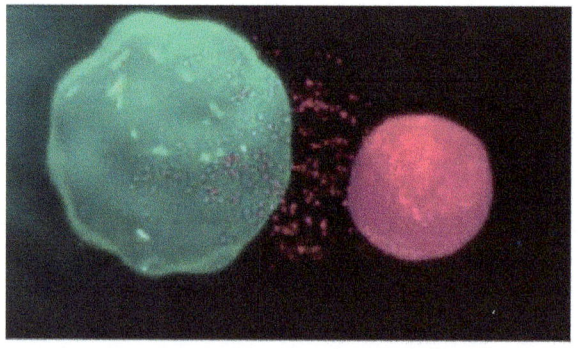

Pus is a thick, often discolored fluid composed of dead tissue, immune cells, and bacteria. It is the body's natural response when fighting off an infection, typically one caused by bacteria.

The appearance and odor of pus can vary based on the location and severity of the infection. It may be white, yellow, green, or brown, and in some cases, it emits a foul smell. Its formation signals the body's ongoing immune response.

Uncovering the Root Causes of Dialysis Needs

Why Pus Forms

Pus usually results from infections where bacteria or fungi enter the body, through the skin, the respiratory system, or mucous membranes. Common entry points include cuts, inhaled droplets, or poorly sanitized surfaces. Poor hygiene can increase susceptibility.

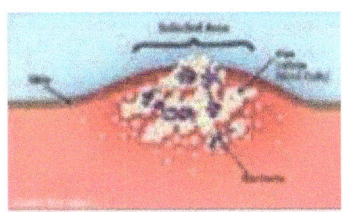

Once the body detects an infection, it triggers an immune response. White blood cells, specifically neutrophils, are sent to the infection site to destroy the invading pathogens. During this battle, many immune cells and tissues die and accumulate, forming pus.

Bacterial strains such as *Streptococcus pyogenes* and *Staphylococcus aureus* are well-known for causing pus-forming infections. These bacteria release toxins that contribute to tissue breakdown, intensifying the infection.

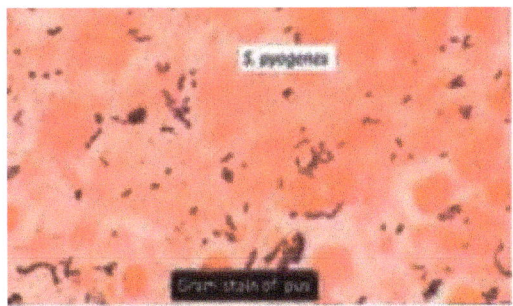

Where Pus Accumulates

Pus commonly collects in a cavity known as an **abscess**, which forms when tissue breaks down. Abscesses may appear externally on the skin or internally within the body.

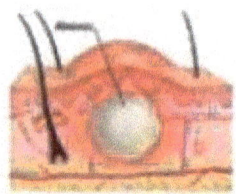

Typical areas where abscesses may form include:

- Skin
- Mouth
- Eyes
- Urinary tract

Body parts that are frequently exposed to environmental contaminants are particularly susceptible.

Symptoms Associated with Pus Formation

When pus forms under the skin, the affected area may become red, swollen, warm to the touch, and painful. These are common signs of a localized skin infection.

In contrast, internal abscesses are more difficult to detect. They may not present visible symptoms but can cause flu-like signs such as

Uncovering the Root Causes of Dialysis Needs

fever, fatigue, and chills. These symptoms can also occur in cases of more severe or systemic infections.

Treating Pus and Infections

Treatment depends on the severity and depth of the infection. For small, surface-level abscesses, a warm compress applied several times a day can help soften the area and encourage the pus to drain naturally.

However, it is crucial **not to squeeze** an abscess. Although it might seem like an easy fix, squeezing can push the pus deeper into the tissue, worsening the infection and creating new openings for bacteria.

For deeper or larger abscesses, medical intervention is necessary. A healthcare professional may drain the pus using a needle or by making a small incision. In some cases, a drainage tube or medicated gauze may be inserted to facilitate healing.

When an infection does not resolve on its own, especially if it is internal or severe, antibiotics may be prescribed. Prompt treatment helps prevent complications and supports the body's natural healing process.

Reducing the Risk of Pus Formation

While some infections are unavoidable, and in such cases, pus formation may be inevitable, there are several precautions you can take to lower the risk and prevent complications.

Start by keeping all cuts, scrapes, and wounds clean and dry. Proper hygiene is crucial. Always use a clean, unused razor, and never share razors with others. Avoid the temptation to pick at pimples, as this can introduce bacteria and increase the risk of infection.

If an abscess does form, it's essential to prevent its spread. This means avoiding the sharing of personal items such as towels, bedding, or clothing that may come into contact with the affected area. Some health experts also recommend temporarily staying away from communal swimming pools or gym equipment that might touch the abscess.

Make it a habit to wash your hands thoroughly after touching any infected area. This simple practice helps reduce the risk of spreading bacteria to other parts of your body, or to others.

It's important to understand that pus is a natural byproduct of the body's immune response to infection. In minor cases, such as small skin infections, pus-filled areas may resolve on their own without the need for medical treatment. However, more severe or persistent infections often require professional care.

In such cases, a doctor may recommend draining the abscess or prescribing antibiotics. If an abscess does not begin to heal or seems to be getting worse, don't wait, seek medical advice promptly to avoid further complications.

6: Clotting Problems and DVT in the Circulatory System

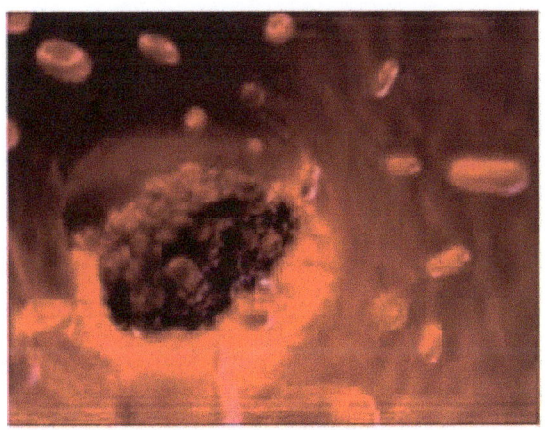

Does Dehydration Spike Blood Sugar?

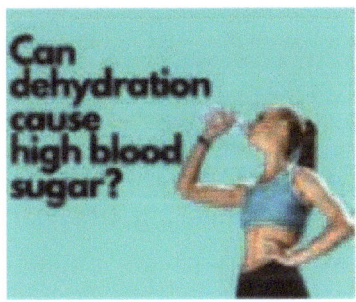

Can dehydration cause high blood sugar?

The short answer is yes, but the mechanism behind it is both fascinating and important to understand, especially for individuals managing diabetes or prediabetes.

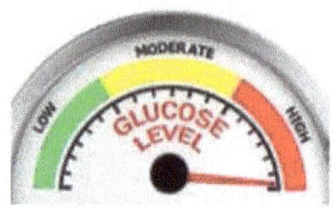

The Physiology Behind It

When you become dehydrated, your body loses more water than it takes in, causing a drop in overall fluid volume, including in the bloodstream. This doesn't change the absolute amount of glucose (sugar) circulating in your blood, but it does reduce the volume of plasma (the liquid part of blood). The result? A more concentrated sugar solution in your veins.

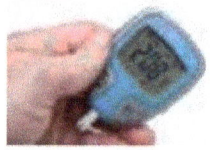

Think of it like making juice from concentrate: if you add less water than recommended, the flavor becomes more intense. Similarly, with dehydration, the "flavor" or concentration of glucose in your blood becomes more potent, effectively raising your blood sugar levels.

A Tasty Analogy: Maple Syrup

To better visualize this, consider the process of making maple syrup. Sap from maple trees is mostly water, about 95%, with just a hint of

Uncovering the Root Causes of Dialysis Needs

sugar. When it's boiled, the water evaporates, leaving behind the thick, sweet syrup we enjoy on pancakes. The sugar content hasn't increased, but it's become much more concentrated due to water loss. That's exactly what happens in your bloodstream during dehydration, except it's not nearly as sweet or harmless.

Why Hydration Matters

Maintaining proper hydration is critical for metabolic balance. Water helps dilute glucose, regulate temperature, support kidney function, and even facilitates insulin transport. When you're dehydrated, not only does blood sugar rise, but your body's ability to process and utilize insulin may be impaired, exacerbating the problem.

The Dangers of Dehydration

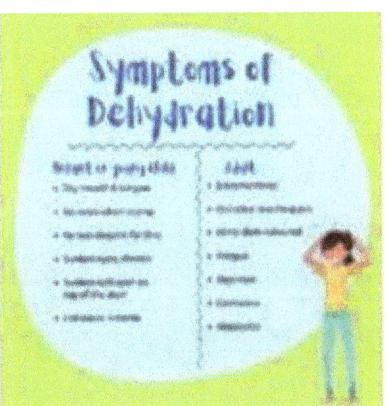

The human body is finely tuned for balance. Even mild dehydration, losing just 1-2% of your body weight in fluids, can affect physical and mental performance, kidney function, and blood sugar regulation.

Factors that often lead to dehydration include:

- **Hot or humid weather**
- **Prolonged physical activity**
- **Illnesses causing vomiting, diarrhea, or fever**
- **Use of diuretics or high-sodium diets**
- **Inadequate water intake during fasting or travel**

In such scenarios, people with diabetes may notice sudden spikes in blood glucose levels, sometimes increasing by **50 to 100 mg/dL** or more. This is especially risky for those on insulin or oral hypoglycemics, as sudden changes in hydration can cause instability in glucose control.

Severe Dehydration: A Medical Emergency

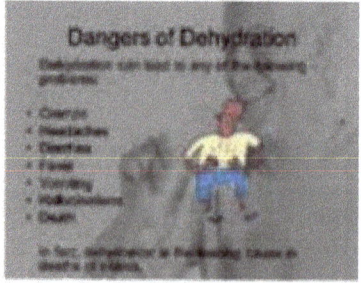

Severe dehydration goes beyond thirst and dry mouth. It can cause rapid heartbeat, dizziness, confusion, and dangerously high blood sugar levels, sometimes leading to **hyperosmolar hyperglycemic state (HHS)**, a life-threatening complication of diabetes. At this stage, the blood becomes thick like syrup, electrolytes are depleted, and organ function begins to falter.

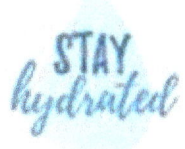

In such emergencies, prompt medical intervention is critical. Rehydration through oral fluids or intravenous (IV) therapy can rapidly bring blood sugar levels down to safer ranges, restore electrolyte balance, and support kidney and heart function.

Caution with Rehydration Drinks

Not all fluids are created equal. While drinks like **Gatorade, Powerade, or Pedialyte** can be helpful in restoring electrolytes, they often contain added sugars that may worsen hyperglycemia if consumed in excess. For those with diabetes, sugar-free electrolyte solutions or plain water with a pinch of salt may be better alternatives, always under medical guidance.

Treating Dehydration Promptly

Dehydration should never be ignored. Chronic or severe cases can contribute to:

- **Diabetic ketoacidosis (DKA)** in type 1 diabetes
- **Kidney damage or failure**
- **Cognitive decline or confusion**
- **Increased risk of heart attacks and strokes**

Monitoring fluid intake and responding to early signs of dehydration, like fatigue, headache, dark urine, or lightheadedness, can prevent these complications before they escalate.

Blood Viscosity and Circulation

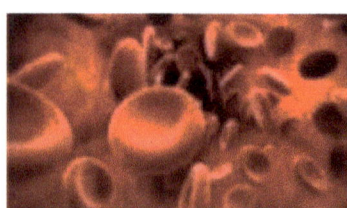

One often-overlooked consequence of high blood sugar is its effect on **blood viscosity**, or how thick and sticky the blood becomes. As glucose concentration rises, so does the "stickiness" of blood, which hampers its ability to flow easily through capillaries and arteries.

Studies have shown that increasing blood glucose levels from 100 to 400 mg/dL can raise blood viscosity by 25% ($\gamma = 0.59$, $p = 0.002$). This increase slows blood flow by around 20% and can elevate blood pressure, placing additional stress on the cardiovascular system.

Other elements that affect blood viscosity include:

Uncovering the Root Causes of Dialysis Needs

- Hematocrit levels (the proportion of red blood cells in the blood)
- Plasma fibrinogen (a protein involved in blood clotting)
- Erythrocyte deformability (the flexibility of red blood cells)

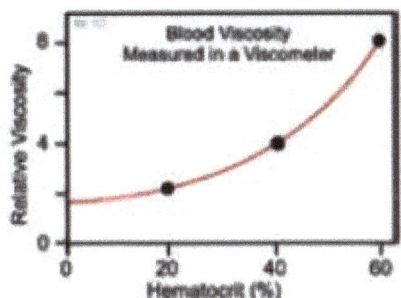

The Role of Plasma Proteins

Plasma viscosity is largely influenced by the concentration of plasma proteins such as:

- Fibrinogen
- Alpha-globulins
- Alpha-2 globulins
- Beta-globulins
- Gamma-globulins

-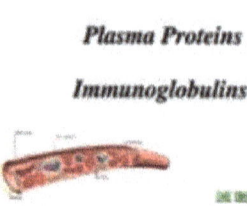

  Plasma Proteins

  Immunoglobulins

An increase in these proteins can cause blood to become more viscous, further complicating circulation.

Hyperviscosity Syndrome (HVS)

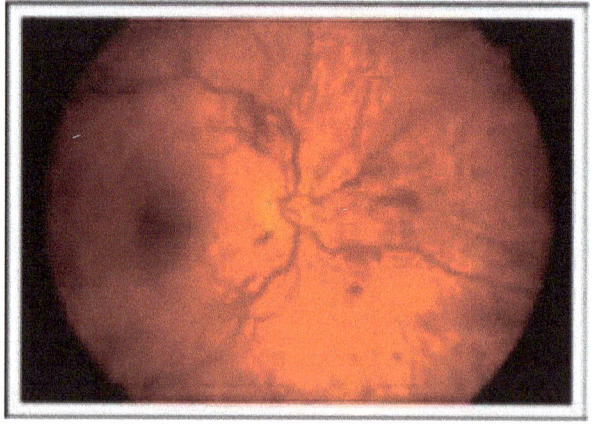

Hyperviscosity Syndrome occurs when blood becomes excessively thick. The symptoms can vary from person to person but often include:

- Dizziness
- Headaches
- Confusion

Uncovering the Root Causes of Dialysis Needs

- Blurred vision

- Shortness of breath

The thickened blood struggles to circulate, especially through the brain and smaller blood vessels. Elevated glucose levels contribute significantly to this condition and can lead to blood vessel damage and clot formation, further burdening the heart and circulatory system.

For more details on how this leads to blood clots, refer to the section on **Hypercoagulability**.

Hypocoagulation: When Blood Fails to Clot Properly

While some conditions cause excessive clotting, **hypocoagulation** is the opposite, when blood fails to clot as it should. This is a serious condition that can lead to dangerous internal bleeding, including in the brain or gastrointestinal tract.

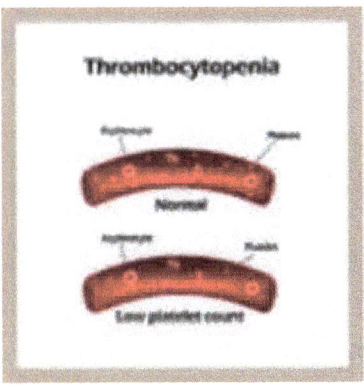

Hypocoagulation may be caused by:

- **Thrombocytopenia** (low platelet count)
- Other disorders that interfere with the blood's ability to form clots

Prompt medical diagnosis and intervention are essential to prevent life-threatening consequences.

The Hypercoagulable State

The **hypercoagulable state**, also known as **thrombophilia**, is a condition in which the body has an increased tendency to form blood clots, or thromboses. This heightened risk can result from inherited genetic factors or acquired medical conditions. While clotting is a normal and necessary process that helps heal wounds, problems arise when clots form inappropriately within blood vessels.

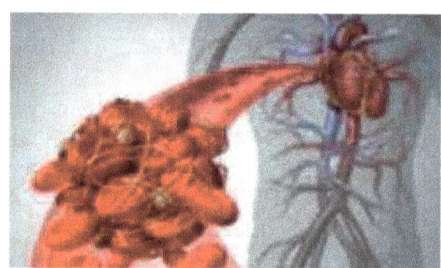

Thromboembolic Conditions and Deep Vein Thrombosis (DVT)

In individuals with a hypercoagulable state, blood clots may develop spontaneously in veins or arteries. This significantly raises the risk of **thromboembolic conditions**, including **deep vein thrombosis**

(DVT) and **pulmonary embolism (PE)**.

DVT typically involves the formation of a clot in the deep veins of the legs or arms, leading to symptoms such as pain and swelling in the affected limb. However, DVT can become more serious if part of the clot breaks away and travels to the lungs, causing a **pulmonary embolism**, a potentially life-threatening event that can impair oxygen exchange and strain the heart.

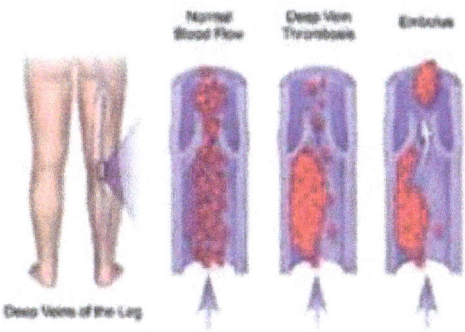

Arterial Clots and Infarction

Clots aren't limited to the venous system. **Arterial clots** can travel to vital organs like the brain, heart, liver, or kidneys. When they block blood flow to these organs, the result is **infarction**, or tissue death due to oxygen deprivation. This may lead to serious complications such as stroke, heart attack, or organ failure, depending on the location of the clot.

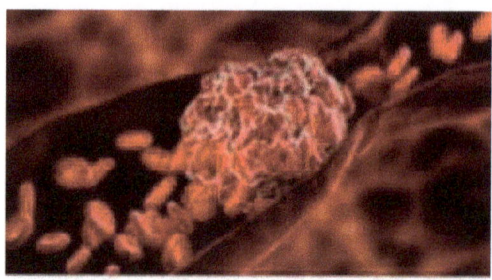

Dehydration and a Possible Link to Insulin Resistance

Emerging research in both animal and human studies points to a close connection between **dehydration** and **impaired glucose regulation**, including an increased risk for **insulin resistance** and **type 2 diabetes**.

When the body is dehydrated (a state referred to as **hypohydration**), it triggers the release of a hormone called **vasopressin**. This hormone instructs the kidneys to retain water to preserve hydration. However, vasopressin also stimulates the liver to produce more glucose, increasing blood sugar levels. Over time, this persistent stimulation contributes to insulin resistance.

People with diabetes are especially vulnerable to the effects of dehydration. When glucose levels rise, the kidneys attempt to remove the excess sugar by producing more urine, which leads to **fluid loss**. Simultaneously, the body may draw water from critical tissues, such as the eyes, muscles, and brain, to maintain internal balance, worsening the effects of dehydration.

Uncovering the Root Causes of Dialysis Needs

The Role of Vasopressin in Blood Sugar Dysregulation

Vasopressin plays a pivotal role in the complex relationship between hydration and blood sugar. When fluid levels in the body drop, vasopressin not only retains water but also stimulates sugar production in the liver. This dual effect leads to **elevated blood glucose** and a gradual loss of insulin sensitivity.

If dehydration becomes chronic or frequent, it may eventually result in **persistent hyperglycemia**, a dangerous condition characterized by consistently high blood sugar levels. Experts emphasize the importance of preventing dehydration, especially for individuals with or at risk of diabetes, to avoid triggering this cascade of metabolic dysfunction.

Treating Dehydration

The good news is that **dehydration is easy and inexpensive to treat**. The most effective remedy is also the simplest: **drink more water**.

However, the amount of water a person needs varies based on several factors, including:

- Gender
- Physical activity levels
- Environmental temperature
- Stress

- Underlying health conditions

It's best to consult a healthcare provider to determine how much water your body specifically requires to function optimally.

DVT: An Overview

Deep vein thrombosis (DVT) is a serious condition involving a blood clot that forms in one or more deep veins, most commonly in the legs. DVT can cause symptoms such as:

- Leg pain

- Swelling

- Warmth or tenderness in the affected area

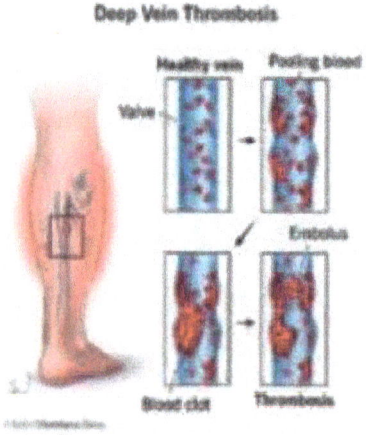

However, some individuals may have **no noticeable symptoms**, making DVT a silent threat. If left undiagnosed or untreated, DVT can lead to **pulmonary embolism**, which can be fatal.

Uncovering the Root Causes of Dialysis Needs

Being aware of DVT and managing risk factors, including dehydration, immobility, or a hypercoagulable state, is essential to protect cardiovascular health.

Individuals may develop **deep vein thrombosis (DVT)** due to underlying medical conditions that affect how the blood clots. A blood clot can also form in the legs when a person remains physically inactive for an extended period. This commonly happens during long-distance travel or prolonged bed rest following surgery, illness, or injury.

When DVT and Pulmonary Embolism Combine

The danger of DVT lies in its potential to escalate. Blood clots formed in the veins can break loose and travel through the bloodstream. If they become lodged in the lungs, they can block blood flow and cause a **pulmonary embolism (PE)**, a life-threatening emergency. When both DVT and pulmonary embolism occur simultaneously, the condition is referred to as **venous thromboembolism (VTE)**.

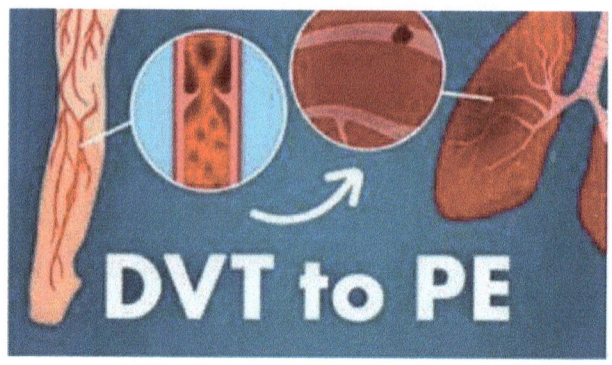

Symptoms and Causes of DVT

Symptoms of DVT may include:

- Swelling in one leg
- Pain or cramping in the affected limb
- Soreness or tenderness
- Skin discoloration
- Warmth in the affected area

However, DVT can also occur **without any visible symptoms**, making it difficult to detect without medical assessment.

The primary cause of DVT is **damage to a vein**, which can result from surgery, inflammation, infection, or trauma.

Uncovering the Root Causes of Dialysis Needs

Risk Factors for DVT

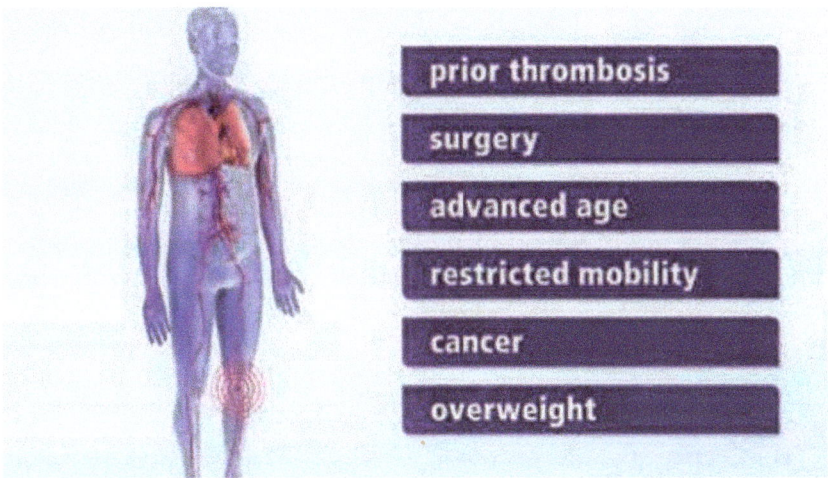

Several factors can increase the risk of developing DVT:

- **Age**: Individuals over 60 are at higher risk, although DVT can occur at any age.

- **Immobility**: Long periods without leg movement, such as during extended travel or prolonged hospitalization, can lead to DVT, especially when the **calf muscles do not contract**, reducing blood flow.

- **Surgery and Injury**: Operations, especially orthopedic surgeries, and physical trauma increase clotting risk.

- **Pregnancy**: Increased pressure in the pelvic and leg veins raises the risk of DVT during pregnancy and up to six months postpartum.

- **Obesity**: Being overweight increases pressure in the veins.

- **Hormonal Therapies**: Use of **birth control pills** or **hormone replacement therapy** raises the risk.

- **Smoking**: Smoking damages blood vessels and contributes to clot formation.

- **Cancer**: Certain cancers release substances that increase clotting potential.

- **Heart Failure**: The heart and lungs work less efficiently in such patients, so even a minor PE can cause severe complications.

Protein C: A Natural Anticoagulant

Protein C is a naturally occurring anticoagulant that plays a vital role in controlling the blood's clotting mechanism. It helps prevent excessive or abnormal clot formation. People who lack sufficient Protein C are more prone to developing dangerous clots because their bodies cannot adequately regulate the clotting process.

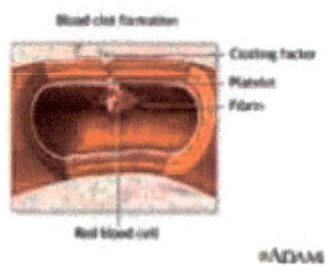

The Role of Protein C and Protein S in Blood Clot Prevention

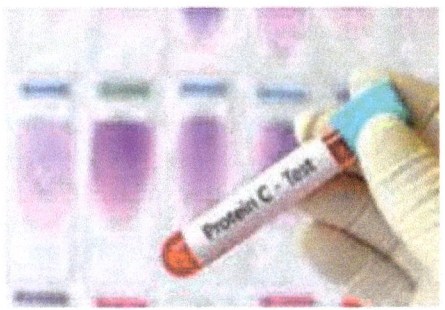

Protein C and Protein S work together to prevent unnecessary clotting. These glycoproteins, synthesized in the liver, are part of the body's natural anticoagulant system and **depend on vitamin K** for proper function.

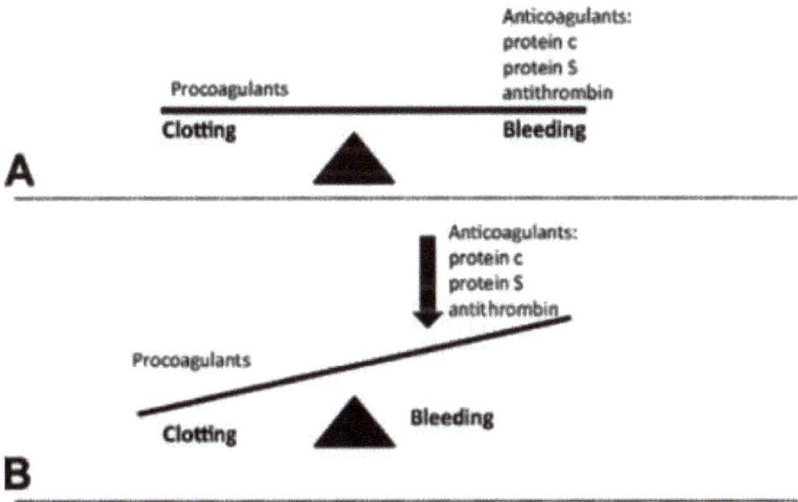

Medical tests can measure the levels and functionality of both proteins to help diagnose abnormal clotting conditions like DVT and PE. A deficiency in either protein can disturb the body's balance between clotting and bleeding, resulting in **unchecked thrombin generation** and a heightened risk of **thromboembolism**.

Natural Blood Thinners Found in Foods

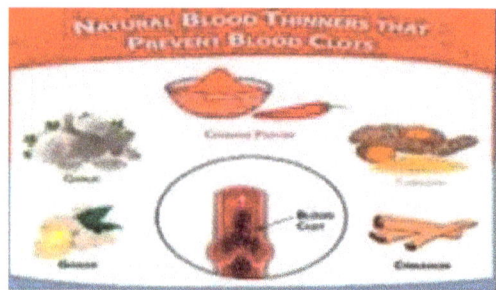

While the body needs to clot blood to heal injuries, **excessive clotting** can lead to complications such as stroke or heart attack. In certain medical conditions, like congenital heart defects, patients may require **blood-thinning medications** to reduce clotting risks.

Fortunately, some **foods act as natural blood thinners**, supporting healthy circulation and reducing clotting risks. These include:

- **Garlic**
- **Ginger**
- **Turmeric**
- **Beetroot**
- **Ginkgo biloba**

Uncovering the Root Causes of Dialysis Needs

- **Leafy green vegetables**
- **Willow bark**
- **Foods rich in salicylates**

While these natural remedies can help, balance is key. **Over-thinning the blood** can lead to complications such as **excessive bleeding** or **anemia**. Therefore, individuals must consult healthcare professionals before making significant dietary or medicinal changes, especially when dealing with clotting disorders.

7: Dialysate Temperature and Ph Balance

Cooling Dialysate – The Benefits

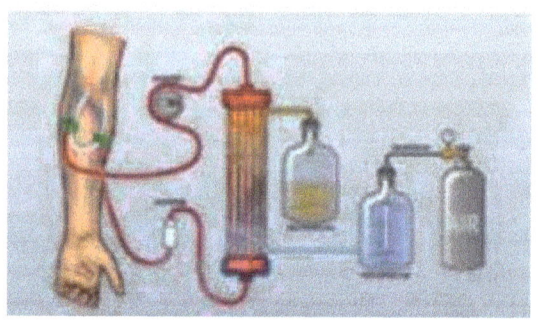

The use of cooled dialysate in hemodialysis isn't a new concept, it has a well-documented clinical history dating back several decades. Initially introduced to induce peripheral vasoconstriction, its primary purpose was to combat a common complication known as intradialytic hypotension (IDH), a sudden drop in blood pressure during dialysis that can cause dizziness, nausea, cramping, and even unconsciousness. Over time, research and clinical observations have built a compelling case for the broader benefits of cooled dialysate, extending far beyond just hemodynamic stability.

A Physiological Rationale

Dialysis, by its very nature, can be a strenuous event for the body. Traditional dialysate temperatures, typically matching core body temperature (~37°C), can lead to **heat transfer** into the patient. This often triggers a cascade of **thermoregulatory responses**, namely vasodilation and sweating, that may further destabilize blood pressure.

Cooled dialysate, usually maintained around 35–36°C (or personalized to be ~0.5°C below a patient's core temperature), helps **prevent this heat accumulation**. The result is:

- Improved **systemic vascular resistance**
- Reduced peripheral vasodilation
- Better maintenance of **blood pressure** during and after dialysis

This controlled mild hypothermia promotes the release of **catecholamines**, like norepinephrine and epinephrine, which naturally encourage vasoconstriction and enhance **cardiac inotropy** (the force of heart contractions), helping stabilize circulatory dynamics throughout treatment.

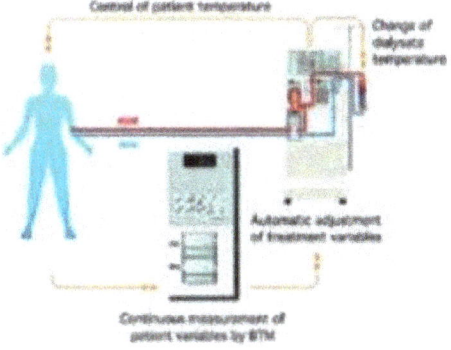

Dialysis Champions

Hemodynamic and Cardiovascular Protection

Numerous clinical trials and observational studies suggest that patients dialyzed with cooled dialysate experience:

- **Fewer episodes of hypotension**
- **Less intradialytic cramping and fatigue**
- **Improved post-dialysis recovery times**

In patients with chronic kidney disease (CKD), who are already at a heightened risk of cardiovascular disease, these benefits are far from trivial. Long-term use of cooled dialysate has been shown to protect the myocardium (heart muscle) by improving left ventricular ejection fraction, and reducing left ventricular mass and end-diastolic volume. These adaptations reduce the workload on the heart and are associated with a lower incidence of cardiac arrhythmias, heart failure, and sudden cardiac death, still among the leading causes of mortality in dialysis patients.

Neuroprotection and Cognitive Benefits

Brain health is another emerging area of interest. During standard dialysis, cerebral perfusion may fluctuate, especially during hypotensive episodes, potentially leading to silent ischemic events or white matter damage over time. The use of cooled dialysate appears to mitigate these fluctuations by enhancing cerebral autoregulation, thereby maintaining more consistent blood flow to the brain. This may help preserve cognitive function and reduce the risk of dialysis-related cognitive decline, an issue increasingly recognized in aging dialysis populations.

Metabolic Efficiency and Toxin Clearance

While the primary goal of dialysis is the removal of uremic toxins and fluid, there has been some concern that lowering dialysate temperature might negatively affect **diffusion rates**, and thus, reduce dialysis efficacy. However, emerging evidence suggests this is not consistently the case.

In fact, some studies have observed:

- Improved urea clearance
- Enhanced overall dialysis adequacy in certain patient populations
- More stable electrolyte balances, particularly potassium and calcium

This may be due to better patient tolerance and longer uninterrupted dialysis sessions when cold dialysate is used, especially in those prone to IDH or fatigue.

At a Glance: Benefits of Cooler Dialysate

- Reduces incidences of intradialytic hypotension
- Enhances hemodynamic stability

- Lowers risk of ischemic brain injuries
- Preserves brain white matter
- Improves cardiac function
- Helps regulate arterial blood pressure during dialysis
- Decreases post-dialysis fatigue
- Boosts patient energy levels
- Maintains dialysis efficiency
- Improves overall health
- Reduces need for nursing interventions during hemodialysis

How Is Cold Dialysis Achieved?

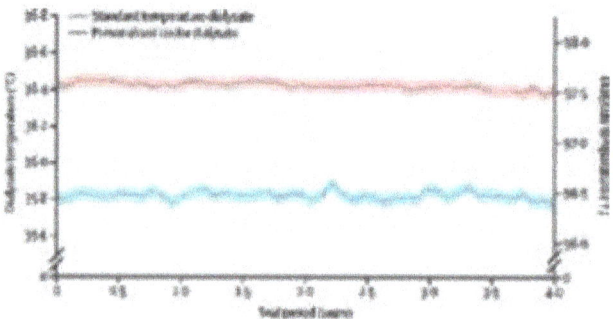

Cold dialysis is implemented by reducing the dialysate temperature to between 35 °C and 36 °C, or approximately 0.5 °C below a patient's resting body temperature. This approach requires no additional costs and can be universally applied. While cooling significantly reduces the risk of IDH and may enhance energy levels, some patients may experience discomfort during treatment.

Maintaining the Body's pH Balance

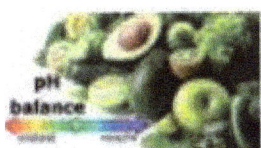

Water is essential to life and has a neutral pH of 7.0. The ideal pH for the human body falls between 7.30 and 7.45. pH, which measures hydrogen ion concentration, is a key indicator of health. When the body becomes too acidic, falling below this optimal range, organs and tissues may be adversely affected.

Acidic conditions in the body can contribute to issues such as acid reflux, heartburn, and inflammation in the digestive tract. Moreover, an acidic internal environment provides a breeding ground for harmful pathogens.

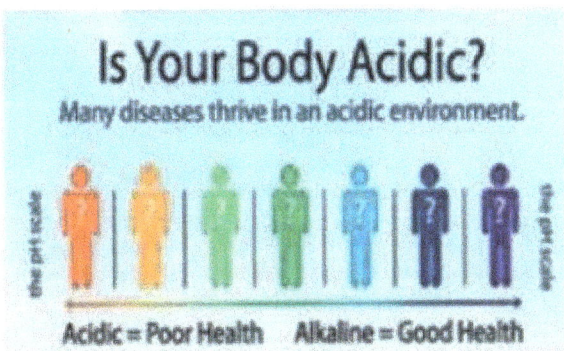

Acid Reflux: An Overview

Acid reflux occurs when stomach acid flows back into the esophagus, often due to an imbalance in body pH. This can cause a burning sensation known as heartburn. While heartburn is a symptom of acid reflux, it is not related to the heart itself.

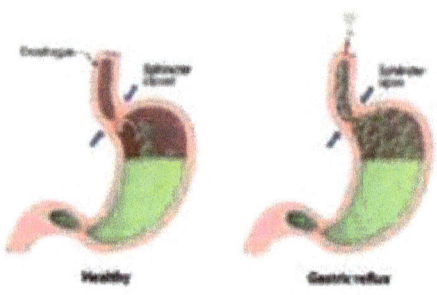

When acid reflux becomes frequent, typically occurring more than twice per week, it may progress to gastroesophageal reflux disease (GERD), a more severe condition that requires medical diagnosis and intervention.

Gastroesophageal reflux disease (GERD) is a common condition, especially in Western countries, affecting roughly 20% of the population. In the United States alone, nearly one in five Americans

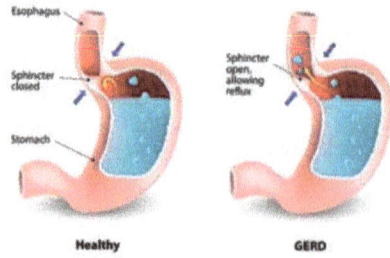

suffers from GERD.

Atherosclerosis and Its Connection with Acidity

Excess acid in the body has been linked to the formation of fatty deposits, or plaques, in the arteries, a condition known as atherosclerosis. Before diving deeper into this topic, it's essential to distinguish between two closely related terms: *atherosclerosis* and *arteriosclerosis*.

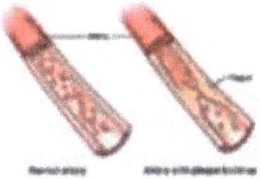

Arteriosclerosis refers broadly to the thickening and stiffening of arteries, the vessels that carry oxygen and nutrients from the heart to the rest of the body. While healthy arteries are elastic and flexible, arteriosclerosis causes them to lose these properties, restricting blood flow to tissues and organs.

Atherosclerosis, a specific type of arteriosclerosis, involves the buildup of fats, cholesterol, and other substances on artery walls. These deposits, called plaques, can also accumulate within the walls of the arteries. Over time, plaques narrow the arterial passage, reducing blood flow. In some cases, plaques may rupture, leading to the formation of blood clots.

Beyond the Heart: Widespread Effects of Atherosclerosis

A common misconception is that atherosclerosis only affects the heart. In reality, it can impact arteries throughout the body. Fortunately, the condition is treatable, and maintaining a healthy lifestyle can significantly reduce the risk of developing it.

Atherosclerosis and Mesenteric Ischemia

When atherosclerosis affects the arteries supplying blood to the intestines, it can cause *mesenteric ischemia*. This condition typically presents as abdominal pain after eating, as the body struggles to deliver enough blood to the digestive system.

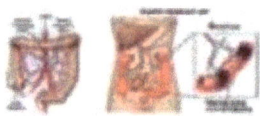

Atherosclerosis and Ischemic Strokes

As acidic conditions in the body contribute to plaque buildup, the risk of blood clots increases. These clots can obstruct blood flow to the brain, leading to *ischemic strokes*, a serious and potentially fatal condition.

Uncovering the Root Causes of Dialysis Needs

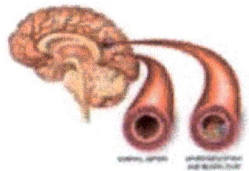

Other warning signs of arterial blockage to the brain include:

- Numbness or weakness in the limbs
- Slurred speech
- Temporary vision loss in one eye

These symptoms may precede a *transient ischemic attack* (TIA), often referred to as a "mini-stroke." If left untreated, a TIA can progress to a full stroke. Additionally, when atherosclerosis affects the coronary arteries, it can result in chest pain, also known as *angina*.

How Is Plaque Formed?

Plaque formation begins with damage to the inner lining of an artery. This damage may result from inflammation or risk factors such as:

- Obesity
- Diabetes
- High blood pressure
- High cholesterol

- Insulin resistance

- Advanced age

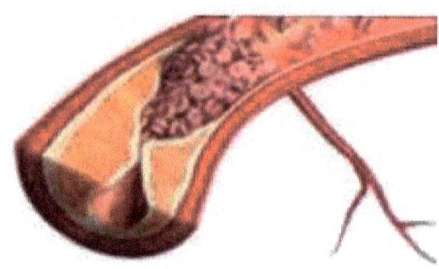

When the artery is injured, the body sends blood components and substances to the site. Over time, fats and cholesterol accumulate, forming plaque. This narrows the artery and restricts blood flow. In some instances, the plaque can rupture, triggering a dangerous blood clot.

Another marker to watch for is *C-reactive protein (CRP)*, which signals inflammation and may indicate an increased risk of atherosclerosis. Other contributors include smoking, sedentary lifestyle, and sleep apnea.

Possible Complications of Atherosclerosis

The complications of atherosclerosis depend largely on which arteries are narrowed or blocked.

Uncovering the Root Causes of Dialysis Needs

If the arteries near the heart are affected, it can lead to **coronary artery disease**. This may cause *angina* (chest pain) or result in a *heart attack*.

When arteries leading to the brain are narrowed, it can cause **carotid artery disease**, which increases the risk of a *transient ischemic attack (TIA)* or a *stroke*.

If atherosclerosis occurs in the arteries supplying the arms and legs, it can cause **peripheral artery disease (PAD)**. PAD is characterized by reduced blood flow to the limbs, making the body less sensitive to temperature changes. This increases the risk of *burns* and *frostbite*. In severe cases, it may lead to *tissue death*, a condition known as *gangrene*.

Another serious complication is the development of **aneurysms**, abnormal bulges in artery walls. Aneurysms can occur anywhere in the body and often develop without symptoms. They may cause localized pain and, if ruptured, lead to life-threatening internal bleeding.

When the arteries that supply the kidneys become narrowed, it reduces the flow of oxygen-rich blood to the organs, resulting in **chronic kidney disease**. Since the kidneys need sufficient blood flow to filter waste and excess fluid, this can severely impair their function.

Preventing Atherosclerosis

Fortunately, atherosclerosis can often be prevented through healthy lifestyle choices. Key preventive measures include:

- Eating a balanced, heart-healthy diet
- Quitting smoking and avoiding smokeless tobacco
- Engaging in regular physical activity
- Maintaining a healthy body weight
- Managing blood pressure, cholesterol, and blood sugar levels

The Connection Between Gout and Uric Acid

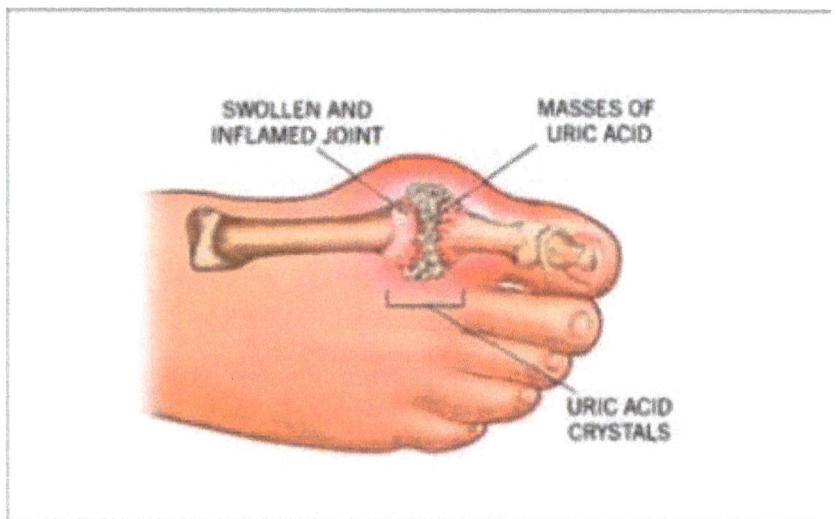

Gout is a form of inflammatory arthritis caused by the accumulation of **uric acid crystals** in the joints. This occurs when blood levels of uric acid become abnormally high, a condition known as *hyperuricemia.*

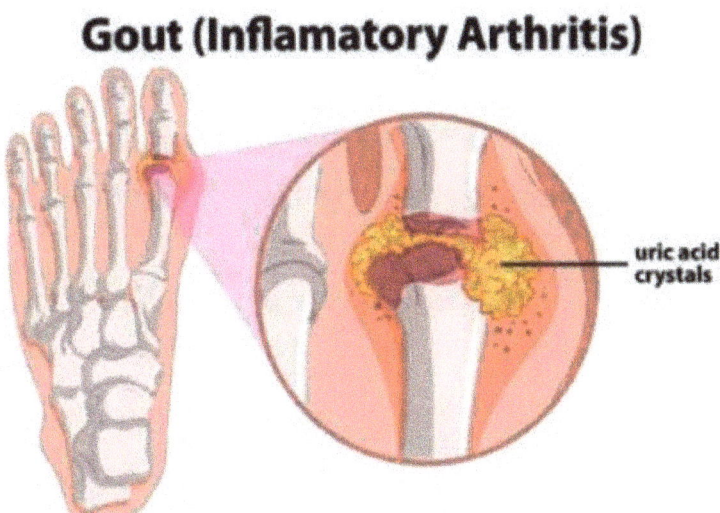

When uric acid crystals build up in the joints, they trigger painful inflammation known as *flares* or *gout attacks*. These episodes can impair movement and significantly impact quality of life. Gout is typically diagnosed when fluid from the affected joint reveals the presence of uric acid crystals.

Treatment usually involves medications to reduce inflammation and relieve pain. In many cases, long-term medication is required to maintain lower uric acid levels in the blood.

How Uric Acid Is Formed

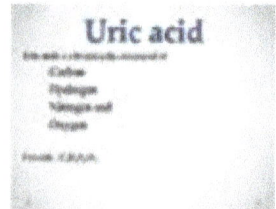

Uric acid is a by-product of the breakdown of **nucleic acids** (DNA and RNA) within cells. As cells naturally die and regenerate, uric acid is released into the bloodstream. It is also formed when the body metabolizes **purines**, chemical compounds found in many foods and beverages. These purines are structural components of DNA and RNA.

Causes of Gout

Gout is more common in **middle-aged men** and typically occurs in **women after menopause**. It often runs in families. Uric acid is primarily removed from the body through the **kidneys**, with a smaller portion excreted via the digestive system.

High uric acid levels can result from the kidneys or gastrointestinal system failing to eliminate it efficiently. Even individuals with normal kidney function may have high levels due to **genetic predisposition**.

Uncovering the Root Causes of Dialysis Needs

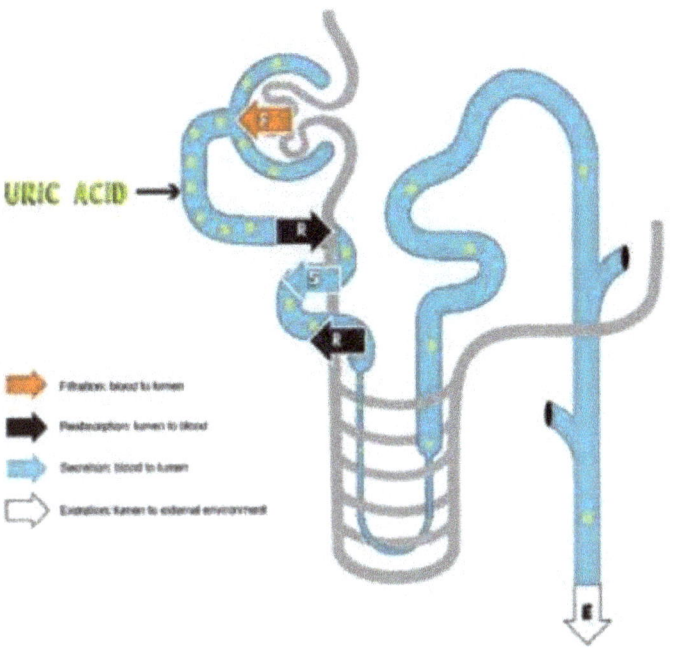

Certain **health conditions**, **medications**, and **toxins**, such as kidney disease, diuretics, or lead poisoning, can impair the kidneys' ability to excrete uric acid.

Diet and Gout

Consuming too many **purine-rich foods** can also elevate uric acid levels. These foods include:

- Red meat
- Organ meats (e.g., liver, kidney)
- Shellfish

- Herring, sardines, mussels

- Asparagus and mushrooms

- Meat gravies

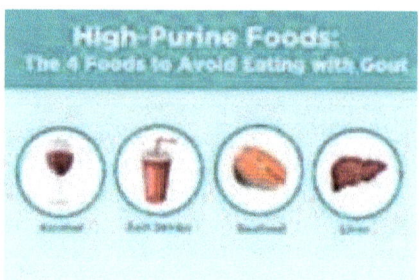

While diet does influence uric acid levels, it is important to note that **dietary restrictions alone typically lower levels only slightly**. A low-purine diet is not a sufficient treatment for those already diagnosed with gout, but it may help as part of a comprehensive management plan.

Patients should also avoid **alcohol** and **high-fructose corn syrup**, both of which can raise uric acid levels and impair kidney function.

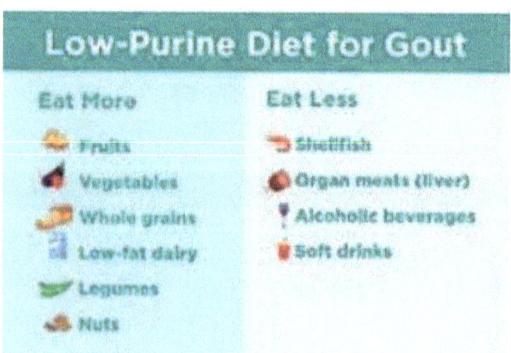

Uncovering the Root Causes of Dialysis Needs

Triggers of Acute Gout Attacks

Acute gouty arthritis can occur suddenly, even without warning. Common triggers include:

- Physical trauma or injury
- Surgery
- Illness or infections
- Certain medications
- Overconsumption of purine-rich foods or alcohol

Cancer and Malignant Cells

Cancer is characterized by the abnormal growth and multiplication of cells. These cells tend to thrive in acidic environments. While many of these abnormal cells eventually die, some adapt by undergoing genetic and metabolic changes, allowing them to survive and evolve into *malignant* cells.

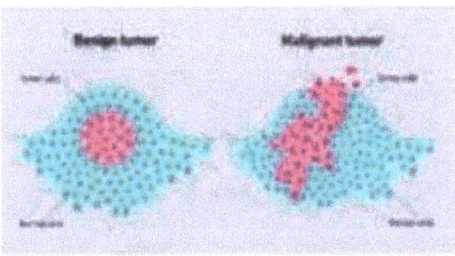

Malignant cells are not typical human cells programmed by normal DNA memory codes. Instead, they originate from a single abnormal cell that has lost its standard growth control mechanisms. These cells divide uncontrollably, invade nearby tissues, and can spread to other parts of the body, a process known as *metastasis*.

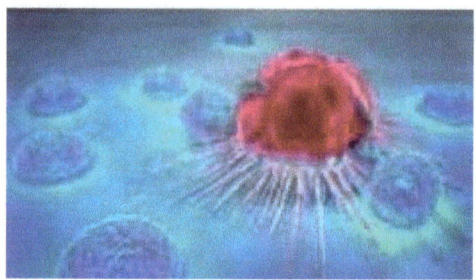

As they migrate, malignant cells stimulate the growth of new blood vessels (a process called *angiogenesis*) to secure a supply of nutrients. These cells can emerge in virtually any tissue or organ in the body.

As cancerous cells continue to grow and multiply, they often form a mass of tissue known as a *tumor*. A tumor is a general term for abnormal cell growth. Tumors can be *benign* (noncancerous) or *malignant* (cancerous). What distinguishes malignant tumors is their ability to invade surrounding tissue and metastasize to distant sites in the body.

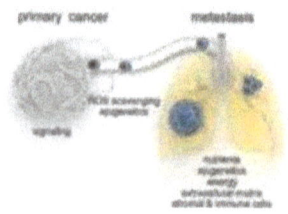

Acid Production by Cancer Cells

As cancer cells proliferate, they increase acid production in the body, which further lowers pH levels and creates a more favorable environment for their survival. This acidic shift can also impair the body's natural ability to maintain a neutral blood pH.

One proposed strategy to counter this involves consuming a *low-acid, alkaline-rich diet*, which may help reduce inflammation and support the body's pH balance. Hydration and intake of alkaline foods are key components of this approach.

Recommended alkaline foods include:

- Apples, blueberries, lemons, grapes
- Soybeans, almonds, wild rice
- Green tea, leafy greens, and other fresh vegetables

Acidic foods to avoid:

- Carbonated beverages, energy drinks
- Popcorn, cheese, and cream cheese
- Pork, red meat, beer, and wine
- Pasta, oats, white bread, and pastries
- Sweetened fruit juices, peanuts, roasted nuts
- Soy milk, barley, and black tea

While dietary strategies alone do not cure cancer, they can complement medical treatments and support overall health.

Cancer Metabolism and the Role of Glucose

Cancer cells rely heavily on glucose for energy production. A key feature of cancer metabolism is a process called *symbiosis*, in which different cancer cells cooperate to sustain survival. In this system, one cell produces ATP (energy) and *lactate* via glycolysis. The neighboring cell then takes up the lactate and uses it to produce ATP through the *TCA cycle* and *oxidative phosphorylation*.

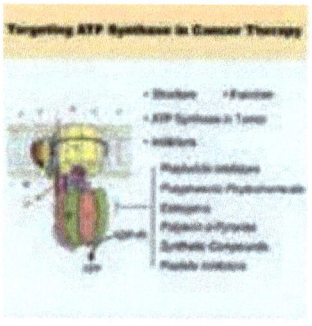

Because cancer cells depend primarily on *glycolysis*, a less efficient but rapid way to generate ATP, cutting off their glucose supply is one proposed way to hinder their growth. Limiting sugar intake may reduce lactate production and ATP generation, making cancer cells more vulnerable.

This also aids the *immune system*, particularly white blood cells responsible for *phagocytosis* (engulfing and destroying abnormal cells), in identifying and eliminating malignant cells.

8: Stroke and HTN

The connection between High Salt Diet, Stroke and HTN

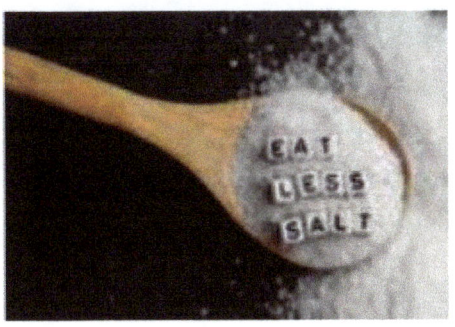

EAT LESS SALT

Your blood pressure and kidneys are more connected than you might think. These bean-shaped organs work tirelessly to filter over 120 quarts of blood every day, removing toxins and excess fluid from the body. But when they are damaged or strained, it's the heart and blood pressure that pay the price.

When everything functions properly, the kidneys filter waste and excess fluid into the bladder to be flushed out through urine. However, a high salt intake makes this task much more difficult. Salt causes the body to retain fluid, making it harder for the kidneys to do their job. As a result, the extra fluid builds up in the bloodstream, increasing blood pressure.

The Impact of Salt on the Heart

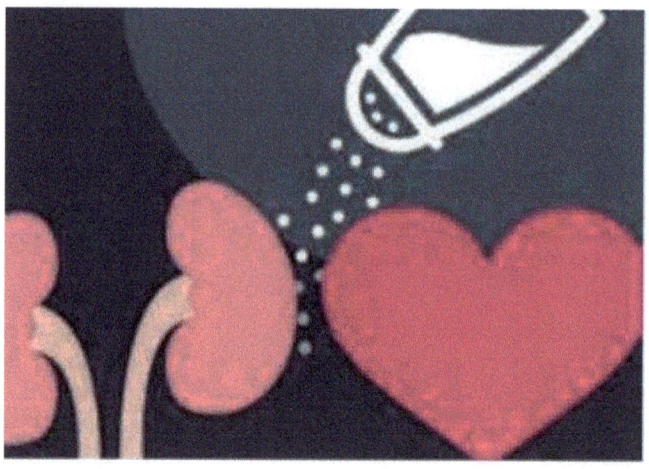

Consuming too much salt over time leads to high blood pressure, also known as hypertension. This condition causes your blood vessels to become stiff and narrow, limiting the flow of blood and oxygen to vital organs.

To compensate, the heart works harder to circulate blood, which raises blood pressure even further. If this continues, it puts immense strain on the heart. The left chamber of the heart begins to enlarge, weakening the heart muscle and eventually leading to heart failure.

Uncontrolled hypertension also damages the inner lining of artery walls. Over time, fatty deposits build up, increasing the risk of heart disease, heart attacks, or strokes. Experts stress that one of the best ways to protect your heart is by preventing damage to your arteries, and reducing salt is a crucial step.

Uncovering the Root Causes of Dialysis Needs

How High Blood Pressure Harms the Kidneys

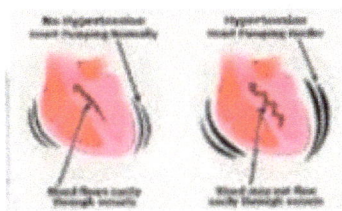

The damage doesn't stop with the heart. High blood pressure also spells trouble for the kidneys. Elevated pressure harms the kidneys' filtering units, causing scarring and reducing their ability to regulate fluids. As this function weakens, blood pressure increases even more, creating a vicious cycle.

If left unchecked, this can lead to chronic kidney disease or even kidney failure. In fact, the two most common causes of kidney disease are hypertension and uncontrolled diabetes.

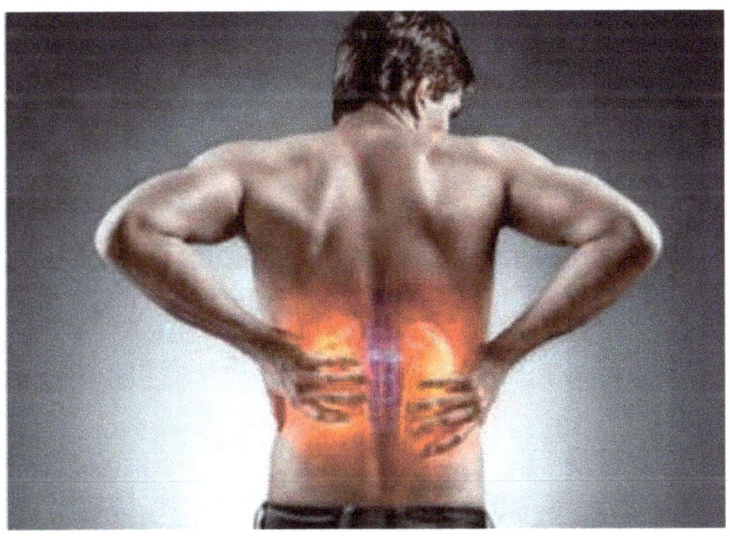

Unfortunately, kidney damage often goes unnoticed until it's advanced. Many early symptoms are subtle or mistaken for other issues. To stay vigilant, watch for the following signs:

- Fatigue
- Difficulty sleeping
- Itchy skin
- Decreased urination
- Blood in urine
- Swelling in the feet, ankles, or around the eyes
- Loss of appetite
- Nausea or vomiting
- Muscle cramps
- Confusion or trouble concentrating
- Metallic or abnormal taste in the mouth

If any of these symptoms occur, especially if you're over 60, have high blood pressure or diabetes, or a family history of kidney failure, seek medical advice from a kidney specialist right away.

Why Salt Affects People Differently

Not everyone reacts to salt the same way. Some individuals can consume sodium with little effect on their blood pressure. Others, known as "salt-sensitive," experience kidney strain and rising blood pressure even with small amounts.

Salt sensitivity is more common among:

- Older adults
- Middle-aged individuals
- People who are obese
- Black individuals

Sensitivity tends to increase with age, so it's essential to monitor salt intake more closely as you grow older.

Lifestyle Changes That Make a Difference

Small changes can have a big impact. To reduce the risk of hypertension and protect your kidneys:

- Follow a low-sodium diet
- Avoid alcohol
- Exercise regularly
- Maintain a healthy weight

That said, lifestyle changes alone may not always bring blood pressure down to safe levels. In such cases, medication may be necessary in addition to healthy habits. These may include:

- **Diuretics (water pills):** Help eliminate excess fluid through

increased urination

- **ACE inhibitors:** Help relax and widen blood vessels
- **Angiotensin II receptor blockers (ARBs):** Also relax blood vessels and lower blood pressure

Lastly, it's a good practice to test kidney function annually, especially if you are managing hypertension or diabetes. Prevention and early detection are key to protecting both your heart and kidneys for the long run.

Understanding the Hidden Dangers of Salt: A Heart and Kidney Perspective

One of the most effective ways to support the long-term health of your heart and kidneys is to consult a medical professional and monitor your salt intake. Even a seemingly small increase in sodium can raise your blood pressure, putting both organs at risk.

Where Most Sodium Comes From

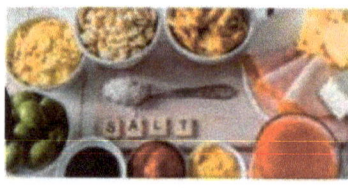

While many Americans assume cutting back on table salt is enough, the truth is more complex. The majority of sodium in the average diet doesn't come from the saltshaker, it comes from processed and packaged foods.

Think canned soups, frozen meals, sauces, deli meats, and snacks.

These everyday items are loaded with hidden sodium. Reducing their consumption can significantly lower your daily sodium intake and, in turn, help prevent hypertension.

What the American Heart Association Recommends

The American Heart Association recommends consuming no more than **2,300 milligrams** of sodium per day. However, the **ideal limit**, especially for individuals with high blood pressure, is **1,500 milligrams** daily.

Research shows that reducing salt intake by just **1,000 milligrams per day** can make a measurable difference in lowering blood pressure and improving heart health.

Common Sources of Sodium You May Overlook

Watch out for these common contributors to excessive sodium:

- Processed and packaged foods
- Naturally salty foods (e.g., seafood, cheese, olives)
- Table salt
- Sea salt and kosher salt
- Over-the-counter medications
- Certain prescription drugs

Even foods marketed as "healthy" can hide high sodium content. Always read labels carefully.

How Salt Alters Blood Pressure: A Quick Overview

Salt is composed of **40% sodium** and **60% chloride**. Sodium plays vital roles in the body, it helps balance fluids and minerals, sends nerve signals, and assists with muscle function. But too much sodium throws this balance off.

When you consume excessive salt, your body retains extra water to dilute the sodium in your bloodstream. This added fluid increases blood volume, which raises blood pressure.

Over time, this sustained pressure can damage artery walls, causing them to stiffen or narrow. This allows **plaque to build up**, eventually blocking blood vessels and increasing the risk of heart attack or stroke.

The result? Bloating, fluid retention, and disrupted fluid balance, all dangerous signs of a system under strain.

Who Is Most Affected?

Some people are more sensitive to salt's effects than others. These factors can heighten salt sensitivity:

- Age
- Ethnicity
- Weight
- Existing health conditions (like kidney disease or

hypertension)

Salt sensitivity means even small amounts of sodium can cause a spike in blood pressure, making salt reduction even more critical for certain populations.

Salt's Impact Beyond the Heart

High salt intake doesn't only burden the heart and kidneys, it affects the entire body. In individuals with elevated blood pressure, the kidneys may begin retaining sodium rather than flushing it out. This fluid retention can cause swollen ankles, fluid around the lungs, and strain on the heart, all signs of worsening health.

The brain is also at risk. Excess salt can damage cerebral arteries and raise the risk of stroke, dementia, and even impair the brain stem, which is responsible for controlling blood pressure and sodium balance.

Emerging research shows that salt can disrupt the immune system as well. High sodium levels affect gut bacteria, leading to inflammation, a precursor to many chronic conditions, including heart disease.

Hemorrhagic Stroke: An Overview

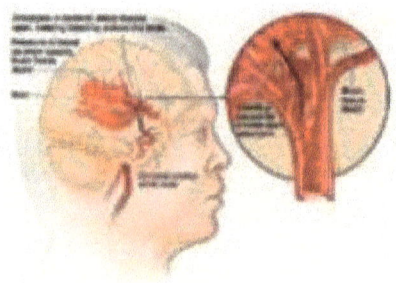

A hemorrhagic stroke occurs when a blood vessel in the brain ruptures, causing sudden bleeding into or around the brain tissue. This bleeding damages brain cells, impairing the function of the body parts controlled by the affected region.

There are two main types of hemorrhagic stroke:

- **Intracerebral hemorrhage**: Bleeding occurs directly within the brain tissue.

- **Subarachnoid hemorrhage**: Bleeding happens in the space between the brain and the thin membranes covering it.

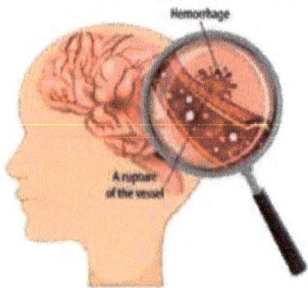

What Happens During a Hemorrhagic Stroke?

A hemorrhagic stroke is essentially a rupture of a weakened blood vessel, resulting in internal bleeding and pressure buildup within the skull. This can cause rapid and widespread damage to the brain unless treated immediately.

Symptoms That Require Urgent Attention

Recognizing the symptoms of a hemorrhagic stroke early can save lives. The faster the treatment, the better the outcome, as fewer brain cells are likely to be permanently damaged.

Common warning signs include:

- Sudden confusion or disorientation
- Sudden numbness or weakness, especially on one side of the body (arm, face, or leg)
- Sudden trouble seeing in one or both eyes
- Difficulty walking
- Dizziness or loss of balance and coordination
- Sudden, severe headache
- Trouble speaking or slurred speech

Other possible symptoms:

- Paralysis on one side of the body

- Light sensitivity
- Stiff neck and neck pain
- Irregular heartbeat
- Breathing difficulties
- Hand tremors
- Trouble swallowing
- A metallic or unusual taste in the mouth

These symptoms should be treated as medical emergencies. Immediate intervention can significantly improve the chances of survival and recovery.

What Causes a Hemorrhagic Stroke?

The most common causes include:

- **High blood pressure (Hypertension)**
- **Head trauma or injury**
- **Cerebral aneurysm** (a weakened blood vessel that bulges and can burst)
- **Arteriovenous malformation (AVM)**
- **Amyloid angiopathy** (a condition where protein builds up in the walls of brain arteries)
- **Bleeding disorders** such as sickle cell anemia

Uncovering the Root Causes of Dialysis Needs

- **Liver disease**
- **Drug abuse**
- **Certain brain diseases**

All of these can weaken blood vessels and increase the risk of sudden bleeding.

How High Blood Pressure Leads to a Heart Attack

High blood pressure places extra strain on artery walls. Over time, this can damage the inner lining of the arteries. Fatty deposits, mainly cholesterol, begin to accumulate, forming plaque in a slow process known as atherosclerosis.

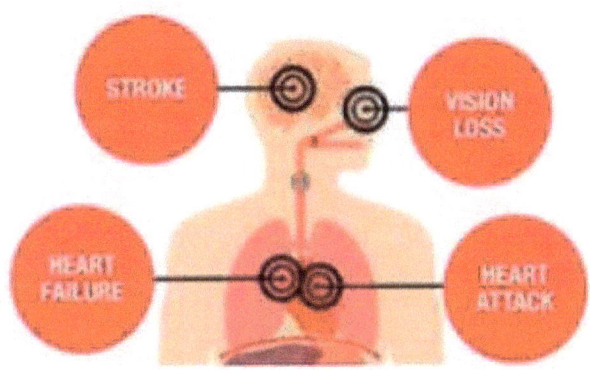

As arteries harden and narrow, the risk of blood clots increases. If a clot or plaque blocks one of the coronary arteries supplying blood to the heart, the heart muscle becomes deprived of oxygen and nutrients. This causes parts of the heart tissue to become damaged or die, a condition known as a heart attack.

Fluid Buildup Around the Heart and Lungs: Pulmonary Edema

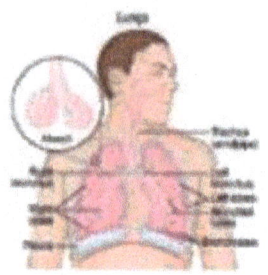

Pulmonary edema is a condition in which fluid collects in the lungs' air sacs (alveoli), making it hard to breathe. While it's often caused by heart issues, there are many possible triggers.

Common causes include:

- **Congestive heart failure (CHF)**
- **Pneumonia**
- **Chest trauma**
- **Certain medications**
- **Exposure to toxins**
- **Strenuous exercise at high altitudes**

Uncovering the Root Causes of Dialysis Needs

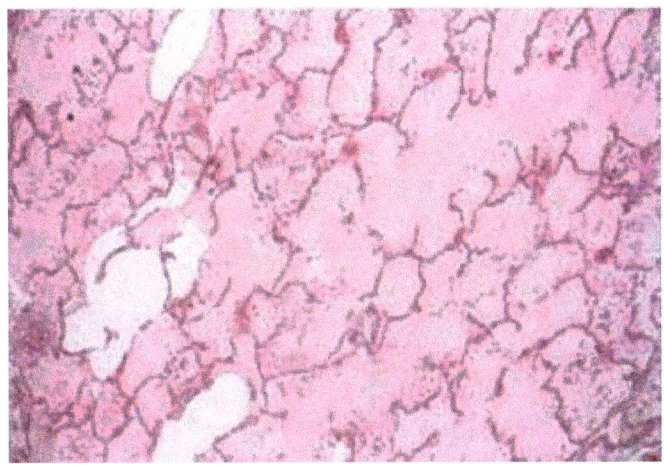

When the heart cannot pump blood efficiently, pressure builds in the blood vessels of the lungs. This forces fluid into the alveoli, preventing normal oxygen exchange and causing **shortness of breath**.

Understanding the Causes of Pulmonary Edema

The most frequent cause is **congestive heart failure**, which may result from:

- A heart attack
- Cardiomyopathy (weakened or stiffened heart muscle)
- Narrowed heart valves (mitral or aortic)
- Sudden spike in blood pressure

Other causes include:

- Kidney failure

- Damage from toxic gas inhalation or severe infections
- Significant physical trauma
- High-altitude exposure
- Artery narrowing to the kidneys
- Side effects of medications

Salt and Its Connection with Calcium Homeostasis and Osteoporosis

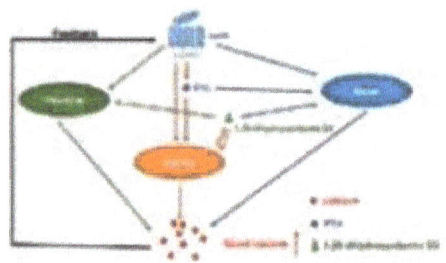

Salt has been identified as a major contributor to increased urinary excretion of calcium. This makes it a significant risk factor for osteoporosis. When sodium intake rises, the body tends to lose more calcium through urine. However, this effect may be mitigated if the intestinal system compensates by enhancing dietary calcium absorption.

Uncovering the Root Causes of Dialysis Needs

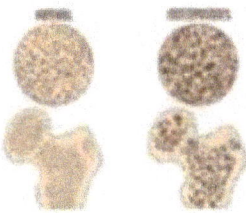

Diets high in sodium are known to disrupt calcium metabolism, primarily by increasing urinary calcium loss, a condition known as *calcinuria* (the presence of calcium salts in urine). As a result, consistently high salt intake elevates the risk of developing osteoporosis.

Calcium Homeostasis: A Hormonal Balance

Calcium homeostasis refers to the body's ability to maintain stable calcium levels. This process is tightly regulated by three primary hormones that manage calcium transport across the gut, bones, and kidneys:

- **Parathyroid hormone (PTH)**
- **1,25-dihydroxy vitamin D_3 (Vitamin D_3)**
- **Calcitonin**

These hormones work in concert to balance calcium absorption, deposition, and excretion.

Salt's Role in Calcium Loss and Bone Health

Salt not only influences calcium levels in the urine but also affects how much calcium is retained in the bones. Because calcium is essential for bone strength, excessive salt intake can lead to calcium depletion in the bones, weakening them and contributing to osteoporosis.

In patients with chronic kidney failure who undergo dialysis, the ability to urinate becomes impaired. As a result, calcium may begin to accumulate in tissues, leading to **calcification**, the hardening of tissues due to calcium deposits.

Understanding Calcification

Calcification refers to the accumulation of calcium in body tissues, which can cause those tissues to harden. While some calcification is a normal part of bodily function, abnormal calcification can be harmful.

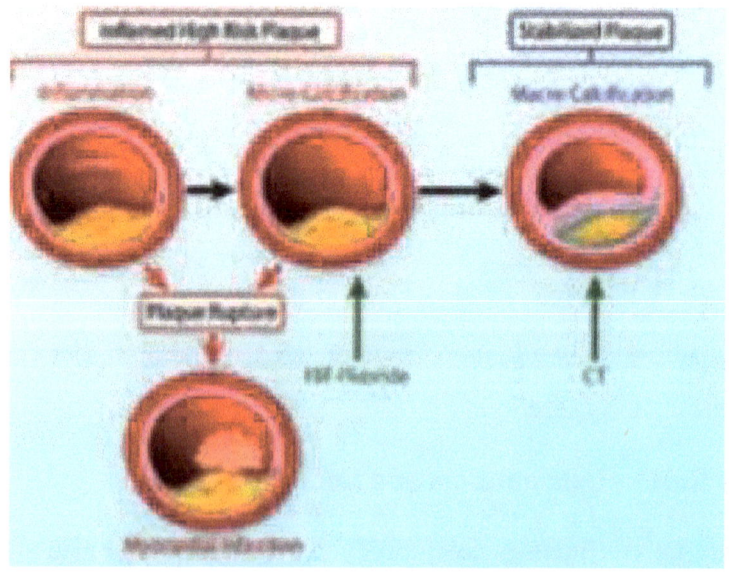

Approximately 99% of the body's calcium is stored in bones and teeth. The remaining 1% circulates in the bloodstream. When this delicate balance is disturbed, often due to certain disorders, calcium may accumulate in soft tissues such as the arteries, brain, kidneys, or lungs. These deposits interfere with normal organ function and are often detectable on X-rays. One common example is calcium buildup in arteries, contributing to **atherosclerosis.**

The Role of Alkalinizers in Reducing Inflammation

Green leafy vegetables, natural *alkalinizers*, are rich in potassium and other vital nutrients. They support vascular health and help reduce inflammation. By doing so, they play a protective role against conditions like **arteriosclerosis** by improving blood vessel function and minimizing calcium-related damage.

9: Lab Values Involved in Dialysis and Assessment Process

Hemodialysis: An Overview

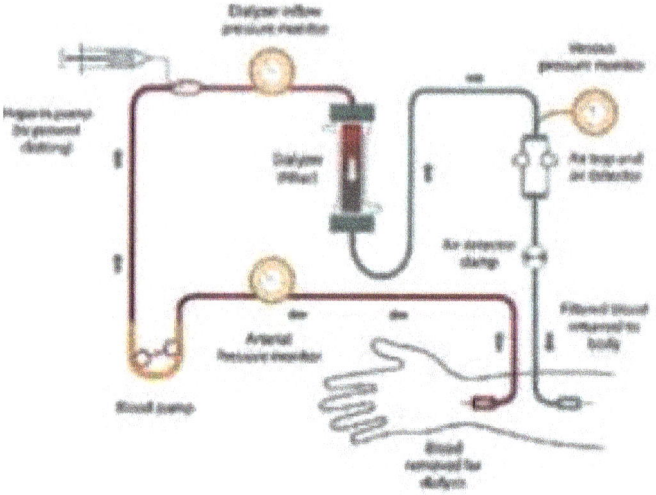

Hemodialysis is a medical procedure in which a machine filters waste products, excess salts, and fluids from the bloodstream, a task typically performed by healthy kidneys. When the kidneys can no longer perform this function adequately, hemodialysis becomes essential. It is an advanced form of treatment for kidney failure that enables patients to maintain an active and healthy life.

Hemodialysis as a Lifelong Responsibility

Hemodialysis must be conducted regularly and executed with precision. For optimal results, patients are expected to follow essential guidelines, starting with taking their prescribed medications on time and consistently. However, the responsibility does not fall solely on the patient.

A specialized healthcare team, consisting of a kidney doctor (nephrologist), a dialysis nurse, and other trained professionals, works closely with the patient to ensure successful treatment. In some cases, hemodialysis can also be performed at home with proper training and equipment.

When Does Hemodialysis Become Necessary?

Hemodialysis becomes necessary when a doctor determines that no other treatment option can adequately support kidney function. Several factors are assessed before making this decision, including:

- The patient's overall health
- Kidney function levels
- Present symptoms
- Quality of life
- The patient's personal preferences

Kidney failure can cause severe symptoms such as nausea, fatigue, vomiting, and swelling. Because these symptoms can escalate quickly, prompt intervention is critical.

One of the most important diagnostic tools is the estimated

glomerular filtration rate (eGFR), which is calculated using blood creatinine levels, age, sex, and other relevant factors. While normal eGFR values vary by age, they are essential for helping doctors decide on the most appropriate treatment plan.

The Critical Role of Hemodialysis

Even in cases of complete kidney failure, hemodialysis allows healthcare providers to manage the patient's blood pressure and maintain proper fluid and mineral balance. This includes regulating essential elements such as sodium and potassium.

It's crucial to begin hemodialysis *before* the kidneys stop functioning completely to avoid life-threatening complications.

Common Causes of Kidney Failure

As discussed in earlier chapters, the most common causes of kidney failure include:

- Diabetes
- Hypertension
- Inherited kidney diseases
- Kidney cysts
- Long-term use of anti-inflammatory drugs

Preparing for Hemodialysis

Uncovering the Root Causes of Dialysis Needs

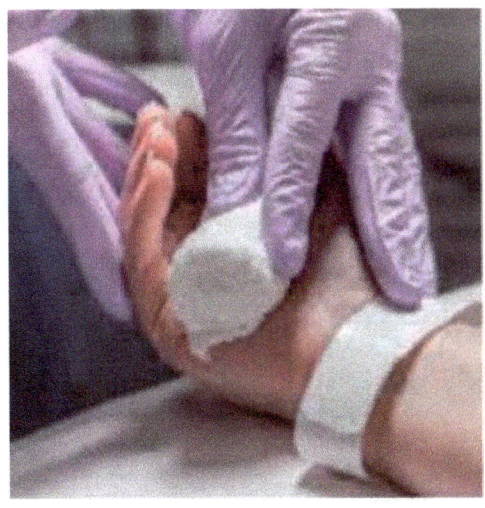

Preparation for hemodialysis should begin several weeks, or even months, before the first session. To begin treatment, the medical team must first establish access to the patient's bloodstream.

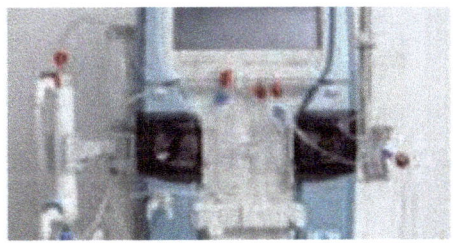

This is achieved by creating **vascular access**, which allows small amounts of blood to be safely removed from the body, filtered through the dialysis machine, and then returned. It is important to note that vascular access sites require time to heal before dialysis can begin.

Types of Vascular Access

There are three main types of access used for hemodialysis:

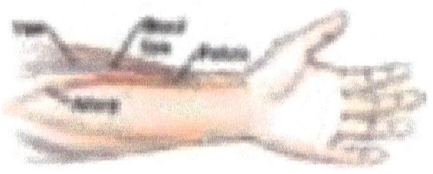

1. **Arteriovenous (AV) Fistula**

    This is the preferred method. A surgeon connects an artery and a vein, usually in the arm, to create the fistula. It is highly effective, long-lasting, and has a lower risk of infection.

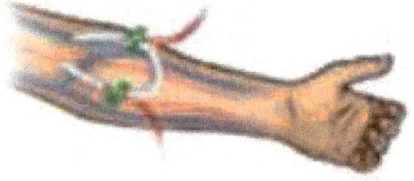

2. **AV Graft**

    If a patient's blood vessels are too small to support a fistula, a synthetic tube (graft) is used to connect an artery and a vein. This method is often chosen when a fistula is not viable.

Uncovering the Root Causes of Dialysis Needs

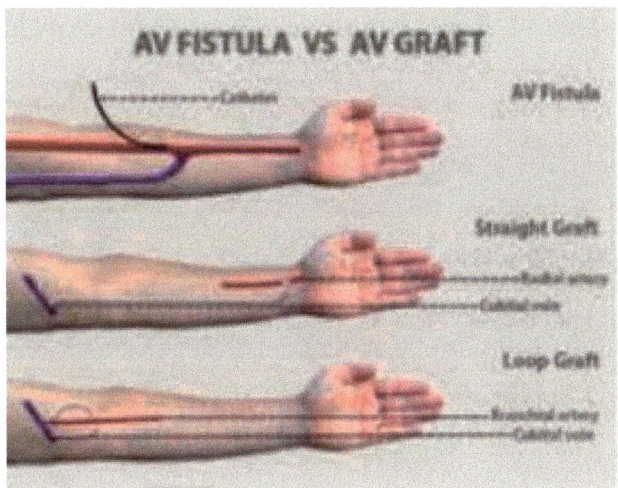

3. **Central Venous Catheter**

In emergency situations or when immediate dialysis is required, a plastic catheter is inserted into a large vein, often in the neck. This access is temporary and carries a higher risk of infection.

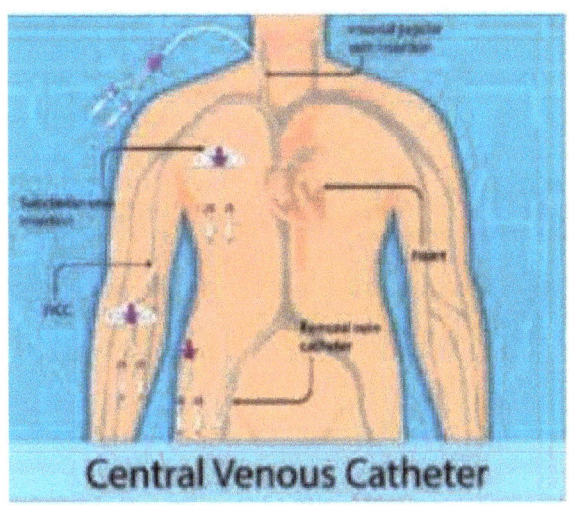

Regardless of the method, careful monitoring and hygiene are essential. Healthcare professionals must diligently care for the access site to prevent infections and other complications.

The Hemodialysis Procedure

During treatment, the patient is seated or reclined comfortably. Blood flows through a dialyzer, a special filter that acts as an artificial kidney. As the blood passes through, waste products and excess fluids are removed before the cleaned blood is returned to the body.

Patients are encouraged to relax during the session. Many choose to watch television, read a book, or take a nap. Those undergoing nighttime dialysis typically sleep throughout the procedure.

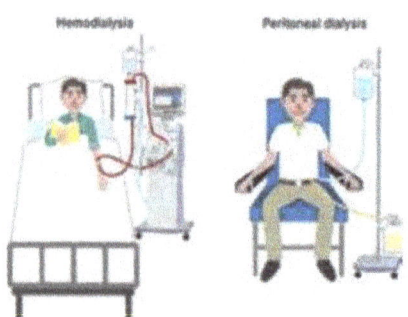

Pre-Dialysis Protocols

Before the procedure begins, the dialysis team carries out a thorough assessment. This includes:

Uncovering the Root Causes of Dialysis Needs

- Recording the patient's weight
- Measuring vital signs such as blood pressure, pulse, and temperature
- Cleaning the skin thoroughly around the access site

This preparation ensures that the procedure is conducted safely and effectively.

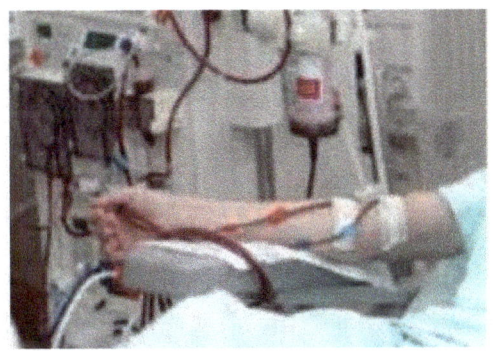

Starting Hemodialysis

At the beginning of the treatment, a surgeon will insert two needles into the patient's arm at the access site. These needles are then secured with medical tape to keep them in place. Each needle is connected to a plastic tube that runs to a machine called a *dialyzer*, which acts as an artificial kidney.

Blood flows through one tube into the dialyzer, a few ounces at a time. Inside the dialyzer, waste products and excess fluids pass into a cleansing solution known as *dialysate*. After the blood is filtered, it returns to the patient's body through the second tube.

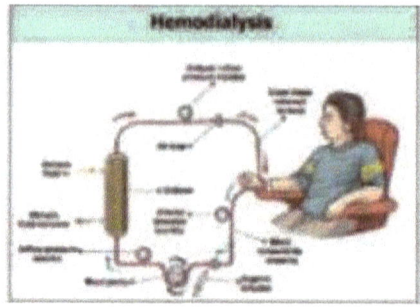

Symptoms During Hemodialysis

Patients may sometimes experience side effects during hemodialysis, including nausea and abdominal cramps. These symptoms often occur when a significant amount of fluid has built up between dialysis sessions and is rapidly removed during treatment.

If a patient becomes uncomfortable during dialysis, healthcare professionals can take several measures to ease the symptoms. This may involve adjusting the rate at which dialysis is performed, modifying the dialysate composition, or changing prescribed medications.

Uncovering the Root Causes of Dialysis Needs

Monitoring During Hemodialysis

> **Monitoring During Dialysis**
> - Vital Signs
>   - Monitor as per your center
> - Monitor the patients behavior, appearance, response and symptoms
> - Give medications as prescribed
> - Monitor the machine for alarms

Close and continuous monitoring is essential throughout the hemodialysis process. Nurses and other healthcare staff regularly check the patient's vital signs, especially blood pressure and heart rate, as these can fluctuate significantly when fluids are removed from the body.

Frequent assessments help ensure the patient's stability and safety during treatment.

After Hemodialysis

Once the session ends, the needles are carefully removed from the access site. A pressure dressing is applied to prevent bleeding and help the site heal. The patient's weight is recorded again to monitor fluid loss during treatment.

Afterward, the patient can resume normal activities until the next scheduled dialysis session.

Results and Importance of Hemodialysis

For patients with *acute kidney injury*, hemodialysis may be temporary and discontinued once the kidneys recover. However, if the kidneys have been severely damaged and show minimal recovery, the patient may require ongoing, lifelong dialysis.

The dialysis team will monitor the patient's treatment progress closely. They ensure that waste products are being adequately removed and will continue to track changes in weight, blood pressure, and overall health.

Monthly Tests for Hemodialysis Patients

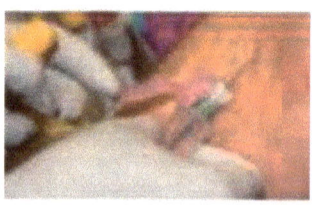

Hemodialysis patients undergo several important tests every month. These tests help assess the effectiveness of treatment and guide adjustments in frequency or intensity:

- **Urea Reduction Ratio (URR):** Measures how much urea is removed during dialysis.
- **Kt/V (Total Urea Clearance):** Evaluates the dialysis session's efficiency in removing waste.

Uncovering the Root Causes of Dialysis Needs

- **Blood Chemistry Panel:** Checks electrolyte levels, mineral balance, and overall metabolic health.

- **Complete Blood Count (CBC):** Assesses red and white blood cells and hemoglobin levels.

- **Vascular Access Flow Measurement:** Ensures proper blood flow through the dialysis access site.

Essential Laboratory Tests Explained

1. **Serum Creatinine**

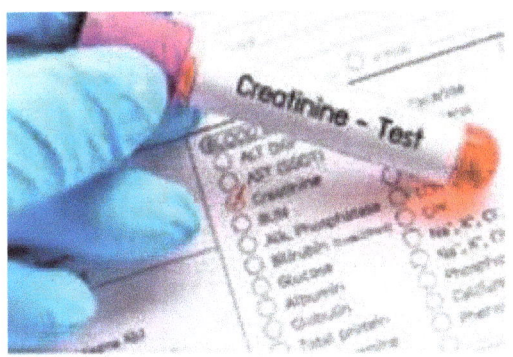

Measures the level of creatinine in the blood, a key marker of kidney function.

- Normal range: 0.8 to 1.4 mg/dL
- Tested during early and late stages of chronic kidney disease (CKD), including end-stage renal disease (ESRD).

2. **Glomerular Filtration Rate (GFR)**

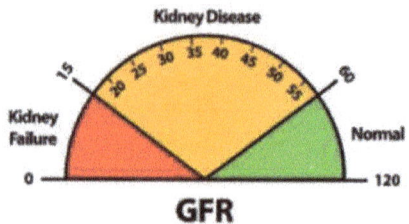

Indicates how well the kidneys are filtering blood.

- Normal: 90+

- Calculated using creatinine levels, age, and gender. A falling GFR signals worsening kidney function.

3. **Microalbumin Test**

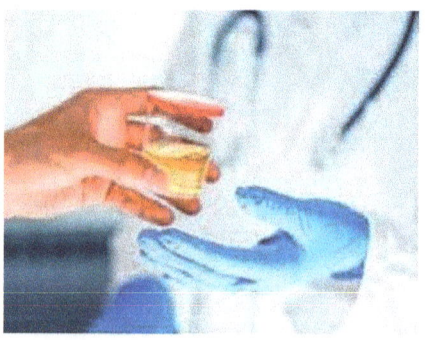

Detects trace amounts of the protein *albumin* in urine, a possible sign of kidney damage.

- Ideal result: No detectable albumin.

4. **Blood Urea Nitrogen (BUN)**

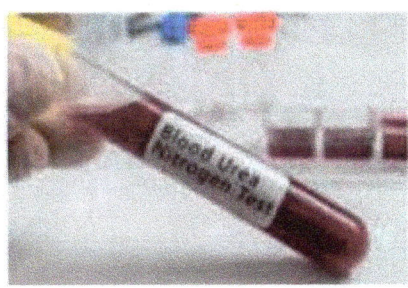

Measures waste levels in the blood to assess how well the kidneys are filtering.

- Normal range: 7 to 20 mg/dL

5. **Creatinine Clearance**

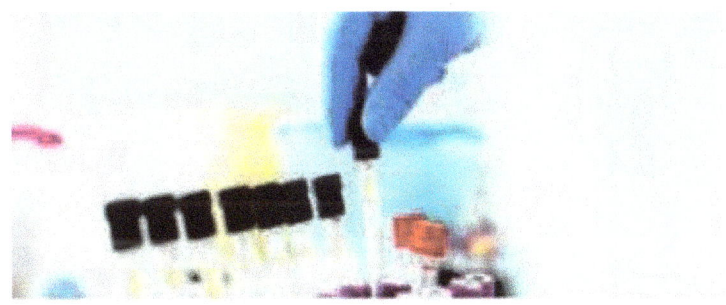

Assesses how efficiently the kidneys are removing creatinine from the body.

- Men: 97 to 137 mL/min
- Women: 88 to 128 mL/min

6. **Hemoglobin (Hb)**

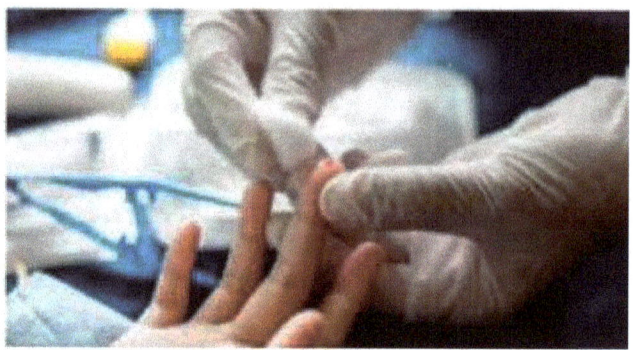

Measures hemoglobin levels in red blood cells and screens for anemia.

- Normal adult range: 12 to 18 g/dL

7. **Hematocrit (Hct)**

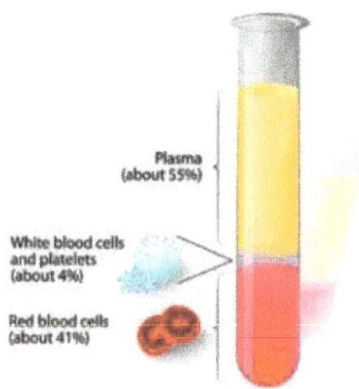

Determines the percentage of red blood cells in the blood.

- Women: 36% to 47%

Uncovering the Root Causes of Dialysis Needs

- Men: 40% to 53%
- For dialysis patients: Recommended range is 33% to 36%

URR – Urea Reduction Ratio

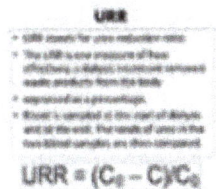

The Urea Reduction Ratio (URR) measures the amount of urea removed from the blood during hemodialysis. A URR of **65% or higher** indicates that the treatment is effectively clearing waste from the bloodstream.

Kt/V

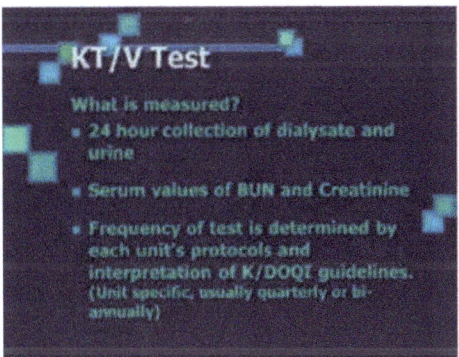

Kt/V is a mathematical formula used to evaluate how efficiently dialysis is removing urea from the blood.

- **K** refers to the *clearance rate*, the amount of urea filtered by the dialyzer.
- **t** stands for the *duration* of the dialysis session.
- **V** represents the *volume of fluid* in the patient's body.

For patients receiving **hemodialysis**, the target Kt/V should be **greater than 1.2**.

For those on **peritoneal dialysis**, the target should be **greater than 2.0**.

This measurement provides a clear assessment of how well the blood is being cleaned during each dialysis session.

A1c – Glycosylated Hemoglobin Test

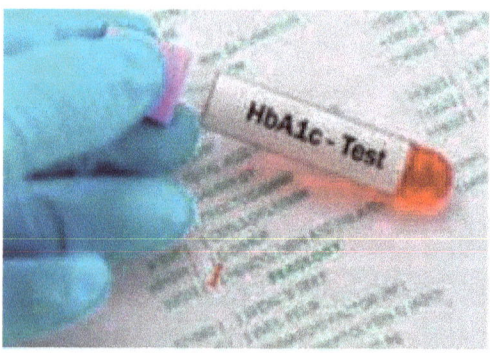

The A1c test, also called Hemoglobin A1c, measures the average blood glucose level over the past **two to three months**. It is primarily used to monitor long-term glucose control in patients with diabetes.

- **Target range:** Less than **7.0 g/dL**

Blood Electrolyte Levels

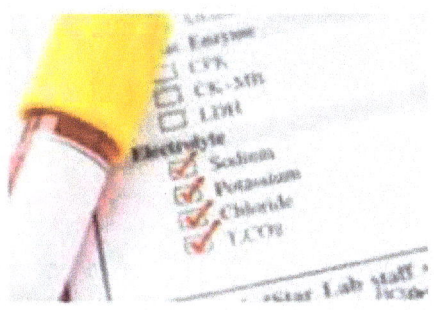

Electrolytes are vital minerals in the body, including sodium, potassium, calcium, magnesium, and phosphorus, that help regulate heart rhythm, fluid balance, nerve signals, and muscle function. Electrolyte testing is especially important for dialysis patients, as imbalances can lead to life-threatening complications such as arrhythmias.

Sodium (Na^+)

Sodium is the body's main extracellular cation and plays a central role in regulating serum osmolality. In dialysis patients, particularly those with severe cardiac failure, managing sodium levels is essential.

Increased sodium levels can improve cardiac function by reducing cellular distance and improving conduction. However, abnormal sodium levels or dysfunction in sodium channels can cause conduction disturbances and contribute to cardiac arrhythmias.

Calcium (Ca^{2+})

Calcium is vital for proper heart function. It regulates the electrical activity of the heart and facilitates the contraction of cardiac muscle cells.

Calcium particles enter heart cells during each beat, helping to coordinate the heartbeat. They also regulate ionic currents and activate myofilaments, promoting healthy heart rhythms and preventing arrhythmias. Impaired calcium movement can disrupt the heart's ability to contract and relax, leading to pump dysfunction.

Potassium (K^+)

Potassium is crucial for cardiovascular health. Low potassium levels can increase the risk of arrhythmia, especially in patients already vulnerable to heart conditions.

It is the main intracellular cation and is essential for maintaining the excitability of the cell membrane. Low serum potassium increases the transmembrane electrochemical gradient, which can impair depolarization and contraction. This may lead to serious rhythm disturbances such as ventricular tachycardia or non-sustained tachyarrhythmias. Potassium levels also influence the effectiveness of antiarrhythmic medications.

Magnesium (Mg^{2+})

Magnesium plays an important role in cellular hydration and works alongside other electrolytes, such as calcium, potassium, and sodium, to maintain fluid balance and cardiac stability.

High serum magnesium levels have been associated with better survival rates in patients with end-stage renal disease (ESRD) and chronic kidney disease (CKD). Magnesium supplementation can help slow CKD progression and reduce the risk of vascular calcification. In some dialysis patients, magnesium may even serve as a safer alternative to albumin for improving outcomes.

Electrolyte Test Overview

The blood electrolyte panel measures the levels of key minerals that help transport nutrients and remove waste from cells. Below are the **normal reference ranges** for each:

- **Sodium:** 135 to 145 mEq/L
- **Potassium:** 3.5 to 5.0 mEq/L
- **Calcium:** 8.5 to 10.5 mg/dL
- **Phosphorus:** 3.0 to 4.5 mg/dL

Maintaining electrolyte balance is critical for dialysis patients to ensure proper heart function, metabolic activity, and overall health.

Post-Dialysis Assessments by Nurses

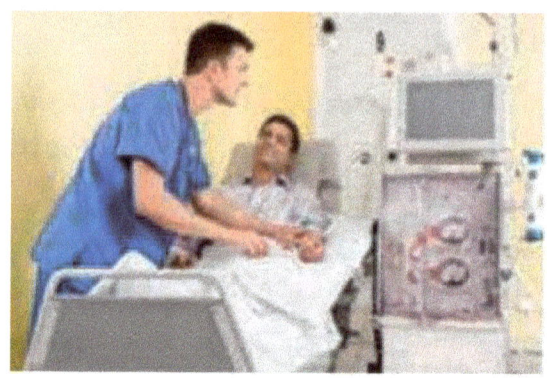

As previously emphasized, dialysis requires careful management even after the procedure concludes. Once a dialysis session is completed, **vascular access** must be thoroughly assessed by the nurse for any signs of bleeding, hematoma, or hemorrhage.

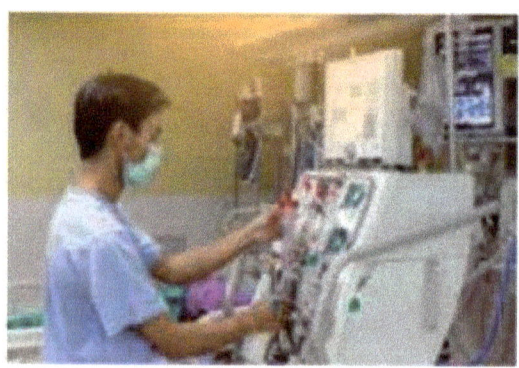

Special attention is needed during patient transfers, from the dialysis center to an ambulance or home. Nurses must ensure **no trauma or pressure** is exerted on the arm where the access site is located. The **vascular site** must be examined for any signs of:

Uncovering the Root Causes of Dialysis Needs

- **Blebs** (ballooning or bulging at the access site)
- **Aneurysms**, which may rupture and cause hemorrhage
- **Infection, redness, or tenderness**
- **Abnormal thrill or bruit**, indicating compromised blood flow

Five Key Indications for Hemodialysis

Nurses must be familiar with the following five major clinical indications to initiate hemodialysis:

1. **Intractable Hyperkalemia** – dangerously high potassium levels unresponsive to medical treatment
2. **Metabolic Acidosis** – persistent low blood pH due to kidney failure
3. **Uremic Symptoms** – such as nausea, fatigue, malaise, and confusion
4. **Therapy-Resistant Fluid Overload** – unmanageable fluid retention affecting cardiac or respiratory status
5. **Chronic Kidney Disease Stage 5 (CKD-5)** – end-stage renal failure

Three Crucial Nursing Diagnoses in Hemodialysis Care

A nurse must plan care for dialysis patients with awareness of the following **priority nursing diagnoses**:

1. **Risk for Injury** – due to altered clotting, blood pressure fluctuations, and vascular access vulnerability
2. **Deficient Fluid Volume** – as a result of rapid fluid removal during dialysis
3. **Excess Fluid Volume** – in cases of missed dialysis sessions or fluid overload between treatments

Common Complications During Hemodialysis

Several **acute complications** can occur during or immediately after hemodialysis. Nurses must be vigilant for the following:

- **Intradialytic Hypotension** – sudden drop in blood pressure during treatment
- **Cardiac Arrhythmias** – due to electrolyte imbalances
- **Dialysis Disequilibrium Syndrome** – rapid shift of fluids and solutes causing cerebral edema and neurological symptoms
- **Allergic Reactions** – to the dialysis membrane or sterilizing agents
- **Bleeding** – especially from the access site
- **Seizures** – associated with severe imbalances or underlying neurological conditions
- **Air Embolism** – rare but potentially fatal complication

Uncovering the Root Causes of Dialysis Needs

The Role of Nephrology Nurses in Hemodialysis

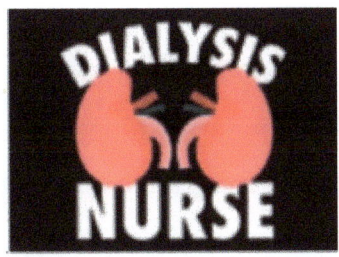

Nephrology nurses are central to the success of dialysis treatment. Their responsibilities encompass clinical, emotional, and educational support for patients with kidney failure.

Registered nurses in dialysis centers are expected to:

- Monitor and record **vital signs** before, during, and after treatment
- **Communicate with patients** to assess their physical and emotional condition
- Provide **education** on kidney disease, treatment options, and lifestyle modifications
- **Answer questions** and address concerns with empathy and accuracy
- **Oversee the dialysis procedure**, ensuring machine settings, timings, and protocols are followed
- **Administer medications** prescribed by physicians
- Monitor for **adverse reactions** to treatment or medications
- Review and interpret **laboratory results** to guide care
- **Report any changes** in the patient's condition to the

Dialysis Champions

nephrologist or supervising physician

10: Common Cause of Death among the Dialysis Patients

The Threat to Dialysis Patients Increased with the Emergence of the Pandemic

End-stage renal disease (ESRD) marks a permanent decline in kidney function, necessitating renal replacement therapy for survival. Although mortality rates among ESRD patients in the U.S. had seen a decline since 2001, the COVID-19 pandemic reversed much of that progress. ESRD patients became especially vulnerable due to their weakened immune systems and multiple comorbidities, placing them at significantly higher risk of both morbidity and mortality.

The Toll of ESRD on the American Population and Economy

As end-stage renal disease (ESRD) continues to rise in prevalence, it places a profound dual burden on the United States, posing a grave public health threat while exacting a growing economic toll. Though remarkable progress has been made since the days when ESRD was nearly always fatal, today's landscape remains fraught with challenges. Advances in medical science have introduced effective maintenance dialysis treatments, enabling patients to live longer and manage the disease. However, in cases of terminal uremia, mortality rates remain unacceptably high.

Despite notable strides in dialysis technology and pharmacological interventions, mortality among dialysis patients is still alarmingly disproportionate. This persistent issue demands urgent attention from both the medical community and policy makers.

Each year, approximately 750,000 Americans are diagnosed with kidney failure. On a global scale, that number exceeds 2 million. The financial burden is equally staggering. Although ESRD patients account for just 1% of those covered by Medicare, they consume roughly 7% of the program's total healthcare expenditures, an imbalance that underscores the disease's enormous cost.

While kidney transplantation remains the most effective long-term solution, it is far from a universally accessible option. Nearly 100,000 individuals are currently on the U.S. kidney transplant waiting list, yet only around 21,000 donor organs become available each year. With the demand growing by nearly 8% annually, the gap between need and supply continues to widen at an alarming rate.

Disproportionate Impact on Minority and Low-Income Populations

ESRD does not affect all Americans equally. The disease disproportionately strikes minority and low-income communities. Data consistently shows that African Americans, Native Americans, and Hispanics experience significantly higher rates of kidney failure compared to their white counterparts. Structural inequalities in

Uncovering the Root Causes of Dialysis Needs

access to healthcare, healthy food options, and preventive care contribute to these disparities.

Mortality outcomes are also unevenly distributed. One year after initiating dialysis, patients face a 15% to 20% mortality rate. Even more sobering is the long-term outlook: fewer than 50% of dialysis patients survive beyond five years of treatment. Age, income level, comorbidities, and accessibility to quality care all heavily influence these outcomes, often to the detriment of already marginalized groups.

Kidney Failure as a Global Crisis: How the U.S. Compares

ESRD is not only an American issue, it is a global health crisis. More than 2 million people worldwide live with kidney failure, and new diagnoses are increasing at a rate of 5% to 7% annually. Countries with the highest prevalence rates include Taiwan, Mexico, the United States, and Belgium.

Though global data on dialysis-related mortality remains limited, earlier studies (such as those from 2007) have revealed a concerning trend: dialysis patients in the U.S. have a 15% higher risk of death compared to their European counterparts and up to a 33% higher risk than patients in Japan. These differences may be linked to variations in healthcare systems, dietary habits, early detection, and patient management strategies.

Currently, approximately 2.5 million individuals with stage 5 chronic kidney disease are dependent on long-term dialysis across the globe. Unfortunately, the outlook for many of these patients is bleak, with annual mortality rates ranging between 10% and 20%. Cardiovascular disease remains the leading cause of death in this population, often exacerbated by the systemic stress of dialysis and underlying metabolic dysfunctions.

Though statins are routinely prescribed to manage cholesterol levels and reduce cardiovascular risk, their effectiveness in lowering mortality rates among dialysis patients has been limited. This raises important questions about treatment strategies and the need for more targeted, disease-specific interventions.

Cardiovascular Prevention to Reduce Mortality in ESRD Patients

Given the strong link between cardiovascular disease and mortality in ESRD patients, lifestyle interventions play a crucial role. The American Heart Association recommends several strategies for cardiovascular prevention, which are applicable to both the general population and dialysis patients:

- Avoid smoking
- Engage in regular physical activity
- Maintain a healthy body mass index (BMI)
- Eat a diet rich in fruits and vegetables

Uncovering the Root Causes of Dialysis Needs

- Include fish in the diet
- Limit salt and sugar intake
- Maintain normal blood pressure
- Control cholesterol levels
- Keep glucose levels within target range

These recommendations help reduce key cardiovascular risk factors such as obesity, high cholesterol, diabetes, and hypertension, all of which are prevalent among patients with kidney failure.

Survival rates for dialysis patients

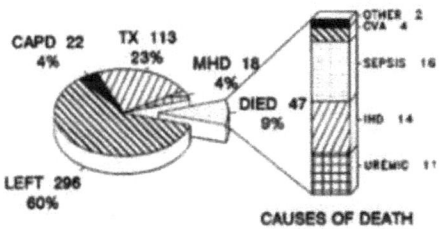

Pie-graph of the distribution percentages of co-morbid conditions that lead to mortality of ESRD

In general, survival rates for dialysis patients are discouraging, with many experts describing them as poor. According to the United States Renal Data System (USRDS), outcomes differ significantly between patients receiving hemodialysis and those on peritoneal dialysis. The three-year survival rate for hemodialysis patients is approximately 57% after the onset of end-stage kidney disease (ESKD), while for peritoneal dialysis patients, it is about 68%. After five years, survival drops to 42% for those on hemodialysis and 52% for those on peritoneal dialysis.

By contrast, deceased donor kidney transplants offer much more favorable outcomes. The three-year survival rate for transplant recipients climbs to 85%, compared to a baseline survival rate of 92–94% for the general population based on age and sex. In fact, the five-year survival of dialysis patients is often comparable to, or even worse than, that of certain cancer patients.

USRDS data also reveal stark life expectancy figures. For patients aged 40–44, the expected lifespan after starting dialysis is approximately 8 years. For those aged 60–64, life expectancy drops to about 4.5 years.

Factors Influencing Dialysis Patient Survival

Several critical factors influence survival outcomes for dialysis patients:

1. Patient Demographics

Age plays a pivotal role in survival rates, with outcomes worsening as age increases. Interestingly, for patients under 45, men tend to have better outcomes than women. However, this trend reverses in patients over 65, where men exhibit a higher adjusted mortality rate.

Race and ethnicity also matter. Studies have shown that Asian Americans and African Americans generally have better survival rates compared to Caucasian patients, although mortality rates vary across different age groups.

2. Dialysis Vintage

Dialysis vintage, the duration a patient has been on dialysis, significantly impacts mortality. Among hemodialysis patients, mortality is highest during the first three months after initiation, a period considered high-risk. It then decreases and reaches its lowest point around the second year, before gradually rising again.

This trend differs for peritoneal dialysis patients, where mortality risk tends to increase steadily after the start of treatment. This pattern highlights the importance of monitoring long-term changes in patient condition and dialysis efficacy.

4. **Dialysis Modality: Hemodialysis vs. Peritoneal Dialysis**

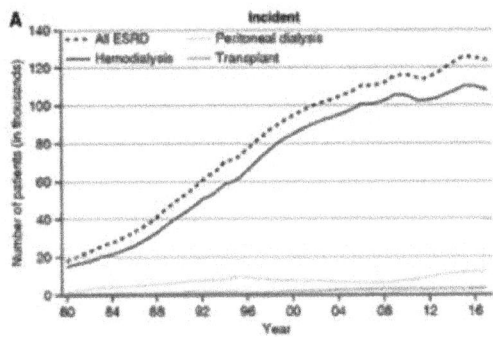

Dialysis Champions

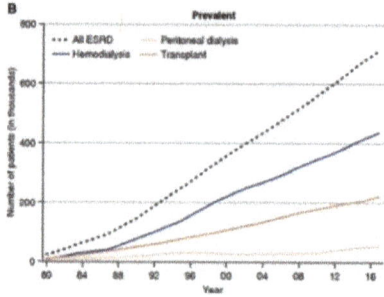

Though detailed comparative data is still developing, existing observational studies suggest that peritoneal dialysis offers better survival rates during the first two years of treatment, likely due to better preservation of residual kidney function. However, after two years, peritoneal dialysis often loses this advantage as ultrafiltration capacity declines.

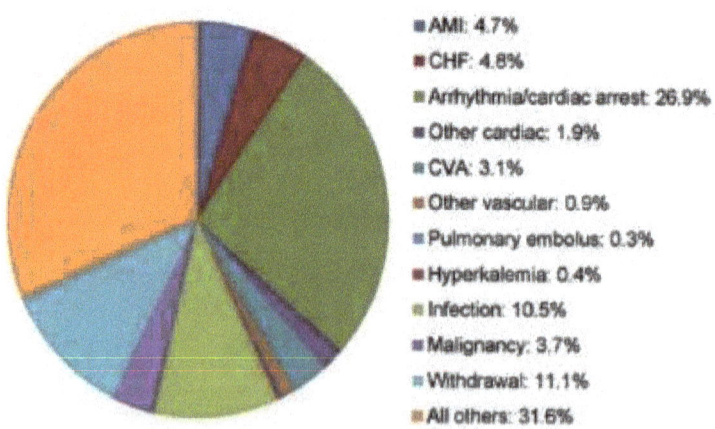

Figure: Arrhythmia and Sudden Death in Hemodialysis Patients: Protocol and Baseline Characteristics of the Monitoring in Dialysis Study

Conversely, patients who start with hemodialysis, often those who are more acutely ill or begin treatment urgently, experience higher early mortality rates. It's also worth noting that hemodialysis is typically used for sicker patients, which may skew survival comparisons between the two modalities.

The Role of Cardiovascular Disease in Dialysis Patient Mortality

Cardiovascular disease (CVD) is the leading cause of death among ESKD patients undergoing dialysis. These patients face a cardiovascular risk far greater than the general population. The most prevalent cardiac condition among them is coronary artery disease.

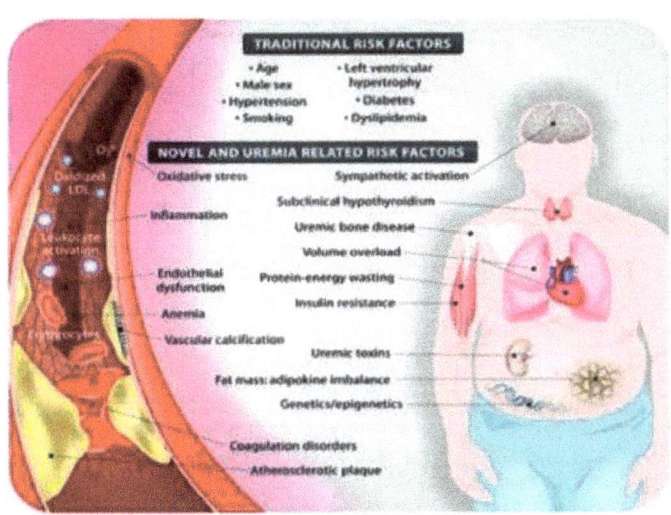

The mortality burden is most severe within the first 120 days of initiating dialysis. Overall, annual mortality hovers around 9%, with a five-year survival rate of only 40–50%. This is 10–20 times higher than mortality rates in the general population.

Effective cardiovascular disease prevention is therefore critical for prolonging life in dialysis patients. Lifestyle recommendations, such as avoiding smoking, maintaining healthy blood pressure and cholesterol levels, and following a balanced diet, can improve outcomes. Infectious complications are the second leading cause of death, while long-term data suggest broadly comparable outcomes between dialysis modalities.

Uremic Pruritus: A Quality-of-Life and Mortality Factor

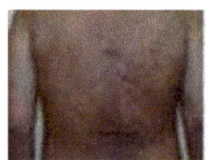

Uremic pruritus is a widespread and often debilitating issue for ESRD patients, especially those on dialysis. Affecting nearly half of all dialysis patients, it is closely associated with poor quality of life and has even been independently linked to higher mortality.

The condition is multifactorial and not yet fully understood, though studies confirm that improving the overall quality of dialysis can reduce both its prevalence and severity. Several treatments have shown promise:

- **Topical and systemic agents**
- **Broadband ultraviolet phototherapy**
- **Gabapentin**, which has been found effective in alleviating symptoms

- **Kappa opioid receptor agonists**, currently under investigation, also show promising results

Although much about uremic pruritus remains unclear, it is increasingly recognized as a significant clinical concern that warrants focused management.

Causes of uremic pruritus

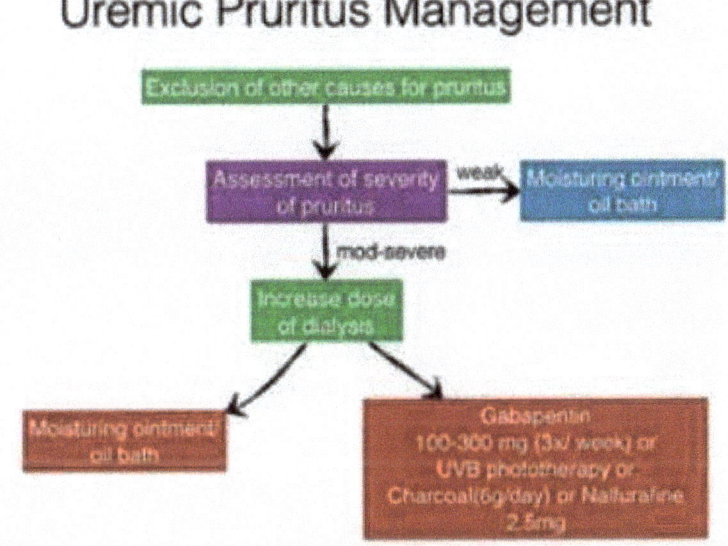

Figure: Uremic Pruritis - Algorithm for Management

Uremic pruritus is a complex and distressing condition commonly affecting patients undergoing maintenance dialysis (MHD). While its exact pathogenesis remains unclear, several triggering factors have been identified. Among the most significant are uremia-related abnormalities involving calcium, phosphorus, and parathyroid hormone metabolism. Additionally, the accumulation of uremic toxins and systemic inflammation are believed to play critical roles in the onset of this condition.

Other contributing factors include **cutaneous xerosis** (abnormally dry skin) and prevalent comorbidities such as **diabetes mellitus** and **viral hepatitis**, which are also recognized as potential triggers.

The Link Between Uremic Pruritus and Mortality

Uremic pruritus is more than just a discomfort, it is a serious clinical complication with significant implications for both quality of life and survival in dialysis patients. Its prevalence among those on maintenance hemodialysis is reported to range widely from 22% to 90%, underscoring its commonality.

Though its multifactorial nature makes it difficult to pinpoint a single cause, research increasingly links uremic pruritus with **systemic inflammation**. This systemic inflammatory response has, in turn, been associated with **cardiovascular mortality** in hemodialysis patients. As previously discussed, cardiovascular disease and infection-related complications remain the leading causes of death in this population.

While large-scale studies specifically examining the correlation between uremic pruritus and mortality are limited, the existing data indicate a meaningful connection. Notably, **severe pruritus** has been associated with higher infection-related mortality compared to patients with milder or no pruritus.

Given this association, **nephrologists and healthcare providers** must exercise increased vigilance in managing cardiovascular and infectious risks in patients experiencing uremic pruritus. Addressing this symptom is not only a matter of improving patient comfort but may also have implications for reducing mortality.

Looking Ahead: Addressing ESRD as a Public Health Priority

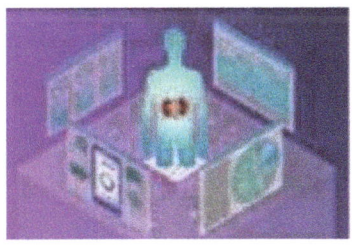

End-stage renal disease (ESRD) continues to pose a significant threat to public health due to its **high morbidity and mortality rates**, along with its substantial **social and financial burden**. Tackling this condition effectively requires a multifaceted approach.

While treatment modalities such as **hemodialysis** and **peritoneal dialysis** are central to disease management, other factors must also be taken into account. These include:

- **Comorbid conditions**
- **Patient age**

Dialysis Champions

- **Duration of dialysis treatment**
- **Supportive care strategies**
- **Implementation of robust infection control protocols**

11: Dialyzable Medications

Medications to Avoid or Adjust Before and During Dialysis

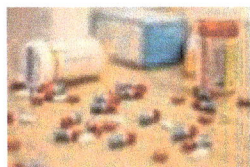
Like other medical procedures, dialysis requires careful consideration of medication management. Certain drugs must be avoided or adjusted before and during dialysis to prevent serious complications. Administering inappropriate medications can pose significant health risks to the patient. Therefore, evaluating and adjusting medication regimens is a critical aspect of dialysis care.

Medications to Avoid During Dialysis

Two major classes of medications often withheld during dialysis include:

- **Blood pressure medications**
- **Certain antibiotics**

Other medications may also need to be withheld depending on individual patient conditions, comorbidities, and the specific dialysis modality used.

Why Some Medications Must Be Held

Dialysis functions as an artificial kidney, filtering and cleansing the blood. However, it may also remove medications from the bloodstream, reducing their effectiveness. In some cases, this could render medications taken before treatment virtually ineffective.

For example, blood pressure medications may need to be withheld before dialysis sessions. This is because they can lead to dangerously low blood pressure during treatment. To prevent hypotensive episodes, healthcare providers often recommend pausing these medications prior to dialysis.

Use of Anticoagulants During Hemodialysis

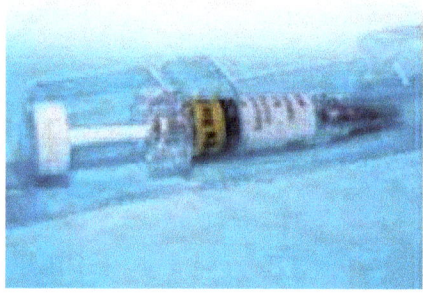

Two primary anticoagulants used during hemodialysis are:

- **Heparin**
- **Enoxaparin**

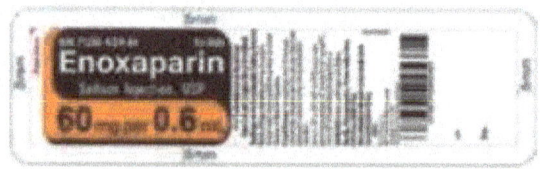

These drugs are essential for preventing blood clotting as blood passes through the dialysis machine. Though often referred to as "blood thinners," anticoagulants do not actually thin the blood.

Instead, they work by **inhibiting Vitamin K-dependent clotting factors** produced in the liver, thereby increasing the time it takes for blood to clot.

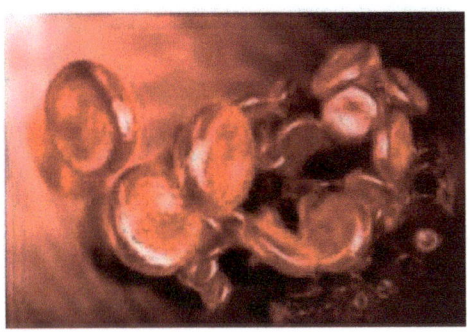

While anticoagulants are effective at preventing the enlargement of existing clots, they **do not dissolve clots** that have already formed.

Drug Interactions and Precautions

Patients on anticoagulants must be monitored for potential drug interactions. Some medications interfere with anticoagulants and may increase the risk of bleeding. These include:

- **Aspirin and other salicylates**
- **Anti-inflammatory medications**, such as corticosteroids and NSAIDs
- **Dextran 40**, used in treating shock
- **Other antithrombotic agents**

Because of the risk of internal bleeding, sometimes without

noticeable symptoms, patients on anticoagulants should avoid contact sports or high-impact activities unless cleared by a physician.

Warning Signs to Report Immediately

Patients should seek medical attention if they experience:

- Difficulty breathing
- Fainting or dizziness
- Hives, blisters, or allergy symptoms
- Prolonged bleeding from minor cuts
- Nosebleeds
- Blood in urine (red or brown color)
- Blurred vision or confusion
- Chest pain or numbness
- Severe abdominal pain or headaches
- Rashes in the mouth or around the eyes
- White or blue discoloration in fingers or toes

These symptoms may indicate adverse reactions or internal bleeding and require prompt evaluation.

Dialyzable Medications: What Does It Mean?

Uncovering the Root Causes of Dialysis Needs

> **What Determines Drug Dialyzability?**
> - molecular size,
> - Protein binding,
> - volume of distribution,
> - water solubility,
> - plasma clearance
> - Dialysis Membrane(Pore size, surface Area)
> - Blood and Dialysate Flow Rates

A drug is considered **dialyzable** if it can pass through the dialysis membrane and be removed from the bloodstream. This is determined by several physicochemical properties of the drug, particularly its **molecular weight**.

- **Low molecular weight drugs** (less than 500 Daltons) are generally removed efficiently during dialysis.
- **High molecular weight drugs** (greater than 2,000 Daltons) are less likely to be removed.

Properties Affecting Drug Dialyzability

Several factors influence whether a drug will be dialyzed:

1. **Molecular Size**

    Smaller molecules pass easily through dialysis membranes,

while larger ones do not.

2. **Protein Binding**

   Drugs bound to plasma proteins form complexes that are too large to cross dialysis membranes. Highly protein-bound drugs are less likely to be removed.

3. **Volume of Distribution (Vd)**

   Drugs with a large Vd are distributed widely in body tissues and are less available in the bloodstream for dialysis clearance.

4. **Water Solubility**

   Drugs with high water solubility are more readily dialyzed. In contrast, drugs with low water solubility or high lipid solubility are removed less efficiently.

5. **Dialysis Membrane and Its Role in Drug Clearance**

   One of the critical components influencing how a drug is cleared during dialysis is the **dialysis membrane** itself. While it has been previously noted that small molecules can pass through this membrane, the dialysis process is influenced by more than just the physiochemical properties of the drug. The membrane's **pore size**, **surface area**, and **geometry** are all key characteristics that determine the extent to which a drug can be dialyzed.

6. Dialysis Flow Rates

Flow rates during dialysis are another essential factor. If a drug concentration in the bloodstream is high, increasing the **dialysate flow rate** may enhance drug clearance. Conversely, when drug concentration is low, a **slower flow rate** might improve removal efficiency. It's also important to note that **the peritoneal membrane used in peritoneal dialysis is larger** than the dialysis membrane used in hemodialysis, which can influence overall filtration dynamics.

Common Dialyzable Medications

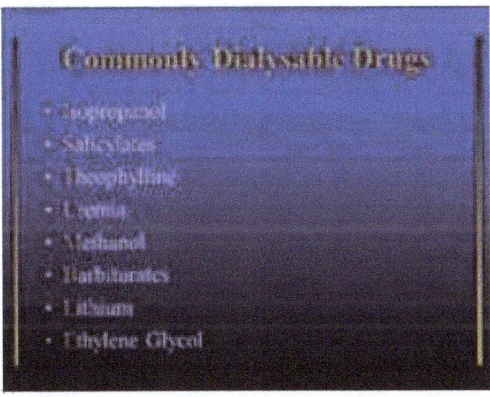

The following medications are commonly removed during dialysis and may require post-treatment re-dosing or alternative management:

- Barbiturates

Dialysis Champions

- Lithium
- Isoniazid (INH)
- Salicylates
- Theophylline / Caffeine (methylxanthines)
- Methanol
- Metformin
- Ethylene glycol
- Depakote (valproic acid)
- Dabigatran
- Carbamazepine
- Isopropyl alcohol

Why Antibiotics Are Given After Dialysis

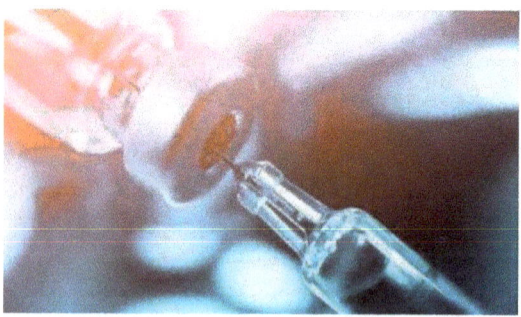

For patients with end-stage renal disease (ESRD), administering intravenous antibiotics **after dialysis** is recommended for several reasons:

Uncovering the Root Causes of Dialysis Needs

1. **Convenience and dosing accuracy** – Post-dialysis administration ensures therapeutic drug levels, as many antibiotics are dialyzable and may be removed during treatment.

2. **Infection prevention** – Dialysis patients are at increased risk of infection due to immune system suppression and the need for vascular access (catheters or needles).

3. **Reduced complications** – Timely antibiotic administration helps avoid thrombotic and catheter-related infections.

4. **Cost-effectiveness** – Prevents the need for additional central venous catheter (CVC) placements, reducing hospital stays and healthcare expenses.

Understanding Dialyzers (Artificial Kidneys)

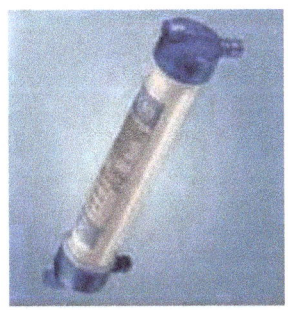

Dialyzers are devices used to filter blood in patients with kidney failure. Each dialyzer contains a **semi-permeable dialysis membrane**, which allows for the **exchange of water and solutes** while separating blood and dialysate.

During treatment, **blood and dialysate flow in opposite directions** on either side of the membrane. This counter-current flow enhances diffusion efficiency and mimics the natural filtration performed by healthy kidneys.

Dialyzer Characteristics

Dialyzer performance is determined by both **design features** and **functional characteristics**.

Design Characteristics:

- Configuration of the dialyzer
- Pre-charge of the blood chamber
- Dialysate chamber
- Type of membrane used
- Biocompatibility of the materials

Functional Characteristics:

These refer to the membrane's **capacity to transfer solutes and water**, a critical measure of dialysis efficiency.

Dialyzer Classification Methods

1. **By Configuration:**
    - **Tube type**
    - **Flat type**
    - **Hollow fiber type** (most commonly used today)

The **hollow fiber dialyzer** contains approximately 8,000–12,000 fibers, each with an internal diameter of 200–300 microns and a wall thickness of 2–30 microns. Blood flows through the fibers, while dialysate flows in the opposite direction outside them. The membrane and casing are sealed with polyurethane for secure filtration.

2. **By Membrane Material:**

    o **Regenerated Cellulose Membranes:** Include copper imitation and cuprammonium membranes. Initially exhibit poor biocompatibility due to free hydroxyl groups, but post-treatment smooths surfaces and enhances compatibility.

    o **Cellulose Acetate Membranes:** Acetylation of the cellulose improves biocompatibility and membrane performance.

    o **Replaced Fiber Membranes:** These use tertiary ammonium compounds to cover hydroxyl groups, offering improved blood compatibility.

    o **Synthetic Fiber Membranes:** Made from materials such as polyacrylonitrile, polymethylmethacrylate, polysulfone, polycarbonate, polyethylene, and polyamide. These membranes offer **high transport and ultrafiltration rates** but are more expensive.

3. **By Ultrafiltration Coefficient (Kuf):**

- **Low Ultrafiltration Dialyzers (Kuf < 15 mL/mmHg/h):**
  Includes copper imitation, cuprammonium, and cellulose acetate membranes.

- **High-Flux/High-Efficiency Dialyzers (Kuf > 15 mL/mmHg/h):**
  These effectively remove **medium and large molecular weight substances**, including β2-microglobulin, making them ideal for patients requiring high clearance of larger toxins.

12: Dialysis Patients Battling with Mental Health Issues

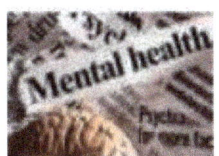

Stress and Kidney Patients: A Closer Look

Stress is a normal part of life, especially for those living with chronic conditions like kidney disease. While occasional stress is manageable, persistently high levels can seriously impact overall health by increasing blood pressure and potentially damaging the kidneys.

But what happens when the kidneys are already impaired? What if the patient is undergoing dialysis? In such cases, managing stress and adopting effective coping strategies becomes critical, not only to maintain well-being but also to prevent further deterioration.

Understanding Stress

Stress can be defined as any physical or psychological factor that disrupts a person's mental and emotional equilibrium. It may arise from physiological triggers such as injury, infection, or illness, or from emotional pressures like anxiety, conflict, or perceived threats.

For individuals diagnosed with kidney disease, the mere

announcement of a chronic condition can be overwhelming, often becoming a significant source of stress in itself.

Stress affects nearly everyone, almost daily. It can stem from both positive and negative life events. Major milestones like marriage or the birth of a child can be stressful, just as much as more difficult experiences like losing a loved one or facing financial hardship.

When the body responds to stress, it triggers a set of automatic reactions, faster breathing, elevated heart rate, tense muscles, and a spike in blood pressure. These responses, part of the "fight or flight" mechanism, are nature's way of helping us navigate immediate threats. However, if these reactions become chronic, the body begins to suffer the consequences.

How Stress Affects Kidney Health

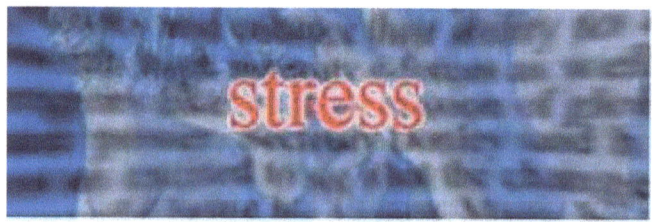

In short bursts, stress can serve as a motivator, pushing individuals to overcome challenges. But when stress becomes prolonged, it no longer helps, it harms. Persistently elevated stress hormones contribute to high blood pressure, increased blood sugar and fat levels, and a heightened risk of chronic diseases like diabetes and heart conditions.

Uncovering the Root Causes of Dialysis Needs

The kidneys are particularly sensitive to changes in blood circulation. When stress raises blood pressure or blood sugar levels over time, the tiny blood vessels and filtration units inside the kidneys can become damaged. People with prolonged high stress are therefore at increased risk for both hypertension and diabetes, two leading causes of kidney disease.

Moreover, stress can exacerbate an already dangerous combination: kidney disease coupled with cardiovascular disease. In such cases, stress can act like a catalyst, intensifying the impact of both conditions. That's why stress management isn't just helpful, it's essential for anyone living with kidney or heart conditions.

Managing Stress: Practical Strategies

Eliminating stress entirely isn't realistic. But learning how to control the body's response to stress can make a world of difference, especially for patients with compromised health.

Here are several tips to help manage stress effectively:

- Eat a balanced, healthy diet
- Limit salt intake
- Reduce caffeine consumption
- Cut down on sugar
- Spend time relaxing or in nature

- Practice relaxation techniques (e.g., meditation, deep breathing)
- Talk to a trusted loved one, friend, or healthcare provider
- Journal your worries and brainstorm solutions
- Set realistic goals and manage expectations
- Aim for 7 to 8 hours of quality sleep
- Maintain a positive outlook
- Take occasional vacations or breaks
- Exercise regularly

Uremic Toxins After Discontinuing Dialysis

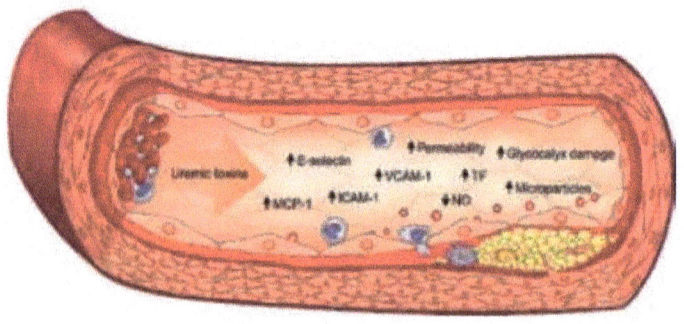

When dialysis is stopped, toxins quickly accumulate in the bloodstream, leading to a condition called **uremia**. As these toxins build up, patients may experience severe symptoms that require medication to manage.

Uncovering the Root Causes of Dialysis Needs

Without dialysis, death typically occurs within days to weeks, depending on how rapidly toxins accumulate. The progression varies from person to person, but the outcome is inevitably the same if treatment is not resumed or replaced with a kidney transplant.

Effects of Uremic Toxins on human body

As toxins accumulate in the body, especially when dialysis is stopped, a person begins to experience a series of physical and emotional changes. Over the course of a few days, the body gradually starts to shut down. Before this final stage, the following symptoms often appear:

- Loss of appetite
- Fluid overload
- Excessive sleeping
- Restlessness
- Disorientation
- Confusion
- Inability to recognize familiar people
- Irregular breathing patterns
- Chest congestion
- Changes in skin color

Medications can help alleviate certain symptoms, such as pain, anxiety, and congestion. Once the body systems shut down, the person becomes unconscious, and the heart eventually stops functioning.

Altered Mental Status Due to High Blood Glucose Levels

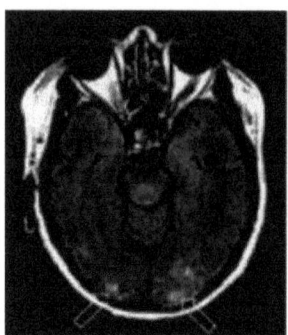

Altered Mental Status (AMS) is a disruption in brain function that causes changes in behavior or awareness. This condition may arise suddenly or develop gradually. Its severity varies, ranging from mild confusion to complete disorientation, sleepiness, or even coma.

Causes of AMS include:

- Low or high blood sugar levels
- Diabetic ketoacidosis
- History of hypertension or diabetes
- Psychiatric conditions

Common signs and symptoms:

- Difficulty concentrating
- Forgetfulness
- Slow reaction times

Uncovering the Root Causes of Dialysis Needs

- Hallucinations
- Changes in sleep patterns
- Agitation
- Reduced or excessive movement
- Rambling or incoherent speech
- Difficulty waking up

Treatment for AMS depends on its underlying cause. It may include oxygen therapy, medications, or hospitalization in severe cases. Some commonly used medications include Hydergine, Haldol, Haloperidol, Fanapt, and Haldol Decanoate.

High Blood Glucose and Infection Risk

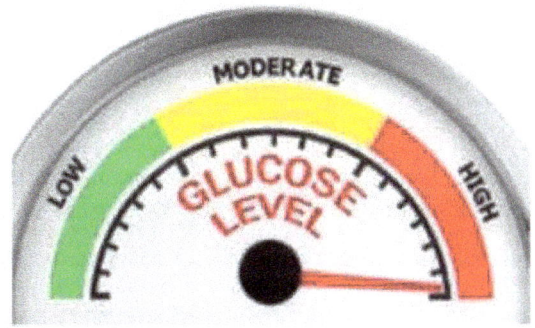

Elevated blood sugar levels impair the body's natural immune defenses, making it more susceptible to various infections, viral, fungal, bacterial, and parasitic. When an infection occurs, it can further raise blood glucose levels, worsening the patient's condition.

Key complications of uncontrolled glucose levels include:

- Weakened immune response
- Increased vulnerability to infections
- Reduced blood circulation, especially in extremities
- Higher risk of diabetic neuropathy

Over time, consistently high blood sugar can cause irreversible damage to the kidneys, eyes, nerves, and blood vessels.

Mental Health Challenges in Dialysis Patients

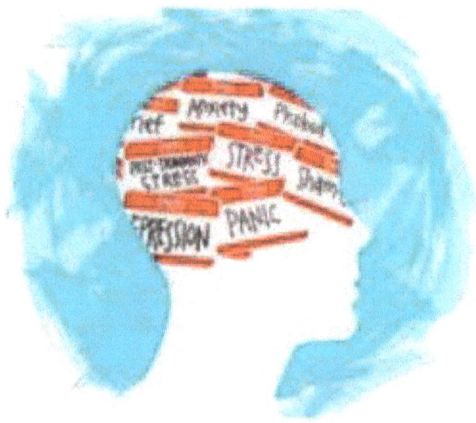

Chronic kidney disease (CKD) is not only a physical illness, it comes with complex psychological challenges. Because of this, a **multidisciplinary care team** is often needed. Mental health professionals work alongside nephrologists to create individualized treatment plans that address both the physical and emotional aspects

Uncovering the Root Causes of Dialysis Needs

of the disease.

Patients undergoing dialysis often show signs of psychological distress. Treatment must be customized, and in many cases, medications and psychotherapy may be necessary.

Dialysis demands absolute reliance on a machine to survive, something no other chronic condition requires to such a degree. This dependency alone has a profound impact on mental health.

Common Mental Health Conditions in Dialysis Patients

Depression

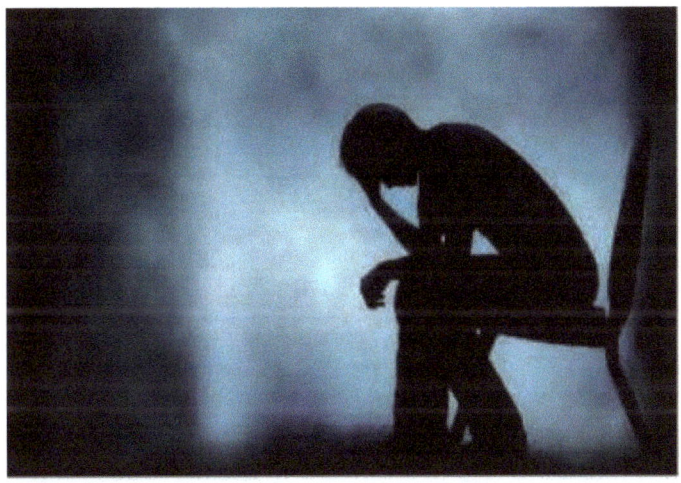

Depression is one of the most frequent psychiatric complications in patients with renal failure. A major contributing factor is the inability of many patients to return to work. Employment not only provides financial security but also offers emotional rewards such as purpose and self-worth. The loss of this role often leads to feelings of inadequacy, hopelessness, and eventually, clinical depression.

Treatment may include antidepressant medication and psychotherapy.

Suicidal Behavior

In severe cases of depression, suicidal ideation becomes a serious risk. Studies have shown that suicide rates are significantly higher in dialysis patients compared to the general population. The consequences of missing even a single dialysis session can be fatal, underscoring the severity of this issue.

Delirium

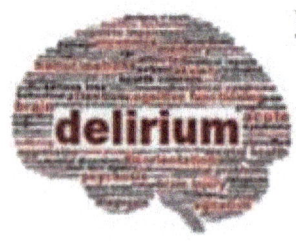

Delirium, especially after dialysis, can result from **electrolyte imbalances**, a condition known as *dialysis disequilibrium syndrome*. Other causes include anemia, uremia, hyperparathyroidism, and complications from medical or surgical procedures.

In elderly dialysis patients, particularly those with diabetes, **dementia** is also a concern. It can arise from various sources, including Alzheimer's disease, dialysis dementia syndrome, or vascular-related conditions.

Mood Swings and Emotional Fluctuations

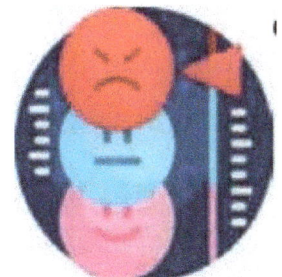

Are mood swings common in kidney patients? Absolutely.

Common causes of mood swings include:

- **Uremia:** Accumulated waste products in the bloodstream can irritate the nervous system, especially early in the diagnosis.

- **Medications:** Many drugs used in treatment can affect mood, sometimes causing depression.

- **Chronic stress:** Living with a life-threatening illness, and being dependent on a machine for survival, is emotionally overwhelming.

Patients often experience a range of difficult emotions, **irritability, anger, frustration, helplessness, and hopelessness**. Without proper emotional support and preparation, these feelings can intensify, worsening both mental and physical health.

The Role of Dialysis Team Members and the Need for Family Support

Ask any renal patient, or those undergoing dialysis, and they will tell you: the journey is filled with emotional, physical, and psychological challenges. The condition demands constant care, and the resulting lifestyle changes can be overwhelming. This burden often extends to the patient's family and loved ones, who also feel the toll of the disease. The situation becomes even more complex when neither the patient nor the family has encountered such a diagnosis before. An unexpected prognosis can increase distress and complicate coping efforts.

In these moments, feelings of helplessness are common. Fear of the future, uncertainty about treatment, and disruptions to everyday life can lead to heightened anxiety for both patients and families. Often, frustration spills over into scrutiny of healthcare providers and the dialysis system. This is where the role of dialysis team members becomes crucial, not just as caregivers, but as compassionate guides and emotional supports.

Dialysis Healthcare Team: Supporting the Patient

Kidney failure is a life-altering condition that requires significant lifestyle adjustments. Tasks that once seemed routine can become daunting. Family members and close friends must step into supportive roles to ease the burden.

Uncovering the Root Causes of Dialysis Needs

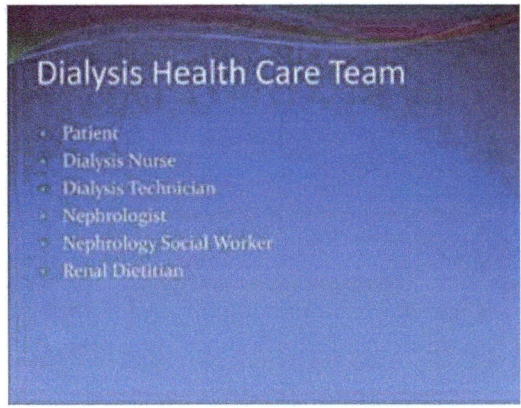

Fortunately, with coordinated care and clear communication, family life can regain a sense of normalcy. Here are some essential steps dialysis teams and families can take to help the patient adjust and reduce stress:

- Discuss concerns openly with dialysis staff, including doctors and nurses
- Write down issues or questions and seek timely solutions
- Ensure dialysis staff keeps family members informed of treatment changes
- Educate yourself using credible resources about kidney disease
- Encourage activities that boost mood and provide emotional relief
- Support the patient in staying active and engaged in daily routines

- Promote regular exercise (as medically appropriate)
- Foster open conversations with trusted friends and family
- Participate in support groups or peer discussions
- Seek assistance from social workers or professional counselors
- Address unresolved family or personal problems proactively
- Adapt treatment schedules around personal goals and priorities
- Be patient and compassionate during adjustments
- Set realistic goals that reflect the new lifestyle
- Consider professional counseling when emotional distress becomes overwhelming

Counseling and Emotional Adjustment

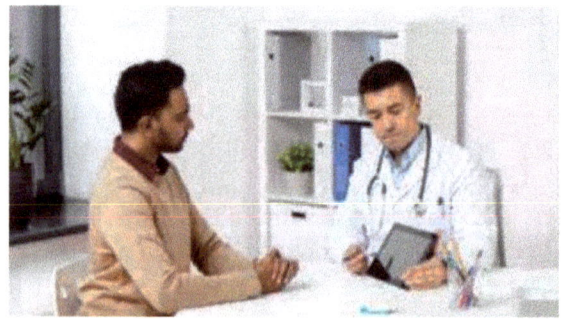

Being diagnosed with kidney disease, and adjusting to dialysis, can be profoundly upsetting, particularly during the initial weeks and months. Patients and their families may experience a form of grief as they learn to accept and manage their new reality. This is a critical time for emotional support.

Most dialysis units include trained counselors or clinical social workers who offer **adjustment counseling**. Professional help should be sought if the patient shows symptoms such as:

- Ongoing depression lasting more than two weeks
- Thoughts of self-harm or suicide
- Significant appetite changes
- Disrupted sleep patterns
- Loss of interest in previously enjoyable activities
- Frequent angry outbursts
- Substance abuse
- Difficulty making decisions
- Social withdrawal

Counseling empowers patients and their families to tap into inner strengths and develop healthier coping strategies. Mental health support from psychiatrists, psychologists, or social workers is not a sign of weakness, it is a vital step toward emotional resilience.

Mental Health Impact of Dialysis and the Role of Nurses

Dialysis Champions

Renal nurses working in dialysis settings often encounter highly stressful and emotionally charged situations. Dialysis patients frequently live under constant psychological strain, which can manifest as frustration or even hostility. Managing these emotional outbursts, while continuing treatment, is critical for both patient safety and the integrity of the healthcare facility.

Nurses are generally trained in the technical aspects of dialysis but often receive limited preparation in managing mental health crises. Because of this, renal nurses must become sharp observers and proactive learners. Their role spans four essential domains:

1. **Ensuring patient and staff safety**
2. **Facilitating holistic, person-centered care**
3. **Educating patients and families**
4. **Providing emotional support**

Challenges Faced by Dialysis Nurses

Despite their dedication, dialysis nurses often face significant obstacles:

- **Patient hostility or severe emotional distress**
- **Lack of formal mental health training**
- **Shortages in staff and specialized personnel**
- **Increased workload due to patient complexity**

Uncovering the Root Causes of Dialysis Needs

To overcome these challenges, institutions must prioritize:

- Mental health education and training for dialysis staff
- Allocating resources to improve staffing and emotional care
- Encouraging collaboration between nurses and other professionals (doctors, counselors, social workers)
- Creating a support system among healthcare team members
- Fostering a culture of confidence and continuous learning

When nurses are better prepared, emotionally, educationally, and professionally, they are more capable of delivering compassionate, effective care. This not only benefits the patient but also enhances the well-being of their families and the healthcare team itself.

13: Delving More into Quality Assessment and Performance Improvement on ESRD

An Overview of Quality Assessment and Performance Improvement in ESRD

It has been nearly 40 years since the End-Stage Renal Disease (ESRD) program was successfully implemented. Over these decades, the program has provided life-saving dialysis therapy to more than 400,000 patients. Like all medical programs, it has undergone continuous evolution, adapting to emerging scientific discoveries and innovations. This adaptability has led to changes in the program's definitions, requirements, and overall goals, especially in response to the shifting demographics and clinical needs of the patient population.

Importantly, the call for reform does not undermine the program's longstanding credibility. On the contrary, the ESRD program has been instrumental in advancing technical aspects of renal care, including the introduction of key medications such as erythropoiesis-stimulating agents and active forms of vitamin D for managing bone disease.

However, as the patient population ages and comorbidities become more complex, new challenges have emerged. The Centers for Medicare & Medicaid Services (CMS) addressed this by issuing the

2008 Final Rule outlining the Conditions for Coverage. This regulation established the dialysis center's medical director as the leader of the interdisciplinary care team, responsible for ensuring the highest standards of quality, safety, and care.

Quality Assessment and Performance Improvement (QAPI)

The QAPI framework places strong emphasis on evidence-based leadership and a culture of continuous learning. At its core, QAPI promotes collaboration between medical directors and dialysis providers to achieve high-quality clinical outcomes. This cooperative approach is vital to optimizing patient health through the delivery of safe, effective, and personalized dialysis care.

The ESRD Quality Incentive Program (QIP)

In 2011, CMS introduced a groundbreaking pay-for-performance initiative: the ESRD Quality Incentive Program (QIP). Designed to link payments directly to performance outcomes, the QIP evaluates facilities based on annually updated quality metrics. Facilities that fail to meet designated performance thresholds face payment reductions.

Success in the QIP requires a comprehensive understanding of its structure, performance metrics, and scoring system. Transparency is a cornerstone of the program, performance data is publicly accessible via facilities and official websites.

With the medical director at the helm, the responsibility for implementing quality initiatives falls squarely on their leadership. They are expected to leverage all available resources to improve patient outcomes, addressing the profound challenges of chronic kidney disease with vision and determination. Both the QAPI and QIP frameworks highlight the critical role of the medical director in driving quality improvements across dialysis centers.

Defining Quality in Dialysis Care

All stakeholders, from healthcare providers to patients and their families, recognize the importance of high-quality care. Nowhere is this more crucial than in the context of chronic illness, where quality of care can mean the difference between life and death.

However, the definition of "quality" in healthcare can vary by institution. In the management of ESRD, quality encompasses not only clinical outcomes but also patient experience, safety protocols, and access to rehabilitative care that supports active living.

Since universal access to dialysis was established nearly 50 years ago in the U.S., the field has seen transformative changes. The original goal of rehabilitation has expanded to encompass a wide array of treatment options, including home-based therapy and large-scale center-based care. These developments have made it possible to treat a growing population of older patients with multiple chronic conditions. The ESRD program has matured to prioritize quality assurance, clinical control, and responsive innovation.

The Evolving Role of the Medical Director

Historically, the medical director's role was limited to providing direct clinical care to the majority of patients in a facility. This began to shift following the 1973 amendments to the Social Security Act, which expanded Medicare coverage for ESRD. The Act required every dialysis facility to appoint a medical director, effectively transitioning the role from individual clinician to team leader.

This broadened the scope of responsibility to include managing a care team composed of nurses, social workers, and dietitians. The medical director became accountable not only for patient care but also for the overall quality of services delivered within the facility.

Medicare ESRD Program and Conditions for Coverage

When the Medicare ESRD program was formalized, the 2008 Conditions for Coverage provided clear guidelines for dialysis centers. These regulations positioned the medical director as the top authority responsible for ensuring compliance with all aspects of care quality.

The responsibilities of the medical director can be grouped into three main areas:

1. **Administrative Duties** – Overseeing operational processes and ensuring regulatory compliance.

2. **Medical Oversight** – Guiding clinical decision-making and patient care strategies.

3. **Technical Expertise** – Supporting the integration of technologies and clinical innovations.

According to CMS, this expanded role is equivalent to a quarter-time position, reflecting its complexity and scope. As clinical challenges grow and healthcare standards evolve, the responsibilities of the medical director continue to expand accordingly.

The Conditions for Coverage (CfC) clearly outline the duties entrusted to the Medical Director of dialysis facilities. While the primary role involves leading the interdisciplinary team, the responsibilities extend well beyond that. The Medical Director is expected to champion individualized patient care and oversee the Quality Assessment and Performance Improvement (QAPI) process.

Core Responsibilities of the Medical Director

Every dialysis facility is required to have a designated Medical Director who plays a pivotal role in ensuring high-quality care. The core responsibilities include:

- Leading the delivery of patient-centered care.
- Driving improvements in patient outcomes.

Uncovering the Root Causes of Dialysis Needs

- Being accountable to the facility's governing body.
- Ensuring the QAPI program functions at an optimal level.
- Overseeing staff education, training, and performance evaluations.
- Developing and updating facility policies and procedures.

The QAPI Program in Detail

Led by the Medical Director, QAPI is a collaborative effort carried out by an interdisciplinary team composed of:

- **Physician** – Usually the Medical Director, responsible for the overall program.
- **Registered Nurse** – Often the clinical manager.
- **Social Worker**
- **Registered Dietitian**

The QAPI team is responsible for fostering effective communication, dedicating sufficient time, and focusing attention on initiatives that enhance patient outcomes. Regular meetings are required, typically monthly or at least quarterly, depending on state laws. All QAPI-related activities, projects, and discussions must be documented.

Key Components of QAPI

The QAPI process follows a structured approach governed by

regulatory expectations, including:

- Developing, maintaining, and evaluating a data-driven quality assessment plan.
- Engaging all team members in the improvement process.
- Adapting the program to match the complexity of services provided.
- Focusing on indicators that reflect improved health outcomes.
- Identifying and reducing errors related to medical practice.
- Documenting evidence of continuous quality improvement.
- Ensuring CMS review and compliance with performance improvement standards.

QAPI Metrics and Focus Areas

To enhance patient health outcomes and minimize medical errors, QAPI employs performance measures and indicators. These include:

- Dialysis adequacy
- Nutritional status
- Mineral metabolism and renal bone disease
- Anemia management

Uncovering the Root Causes of Dialysis Needs

- Vascular access optimization
- Identification of medical injuries and errors
- Oversight of hemodialyzer reuse (where applicable)
- Patient satisfaction and grievance resolution
- Infection control, including:
  - Infection trend analysis and documentation
  - Baseline data development on infection rates
  - Action plan development to reduce infections
  - Promotion of immunizations
  - Preventive strategies to avoid future incidents

A critical part of QAPI is the ongoing monitoring and prioritization of performance improvement activities.

Avoiding the Pitfall of Metric-Driven Mindsets

Recent trends show a growing focus on achieving numeric targets, sometimes at the expense of broader patient-centered care. While achieving benchmarks is essential, it must not come at the cost of overlooking other critical responsibilities and systemic needs.

Rather than concentrating solely on outliers or individual cases that deviate from norms, the Medical Director must guide the facility toward addressing broader quality issues that affect entire patient populations. The success of QAPI hinges on a strategic approach that maximizes improvements for the largest number of patients, ensuring collective rather than isolated progress.

The Medical Director as a Leader in Population Health

True quality improvement goes beyond treating sick individuals who fall short of targets. These cases should still receive focused clinical care, but the QAPI program emphasizes identifying systemic trends, infrastructure issues, gaps in access, and adherence to care plans. These broader insights are essential in understanding why some patients, and sometimes entire cohorts, do not achieve desired outcomes.

To address these challenges, dialysis facilities must be empowered to implement tailored changes that benefit both current and future patients. The Medical Director, in this context, transitions from the traditional role of direct care provider to that of a population health leader, responsible for system-wide quality assurance and sustainable improvements in care delivery.

14: Transforming Lives Through Kidney Transplant

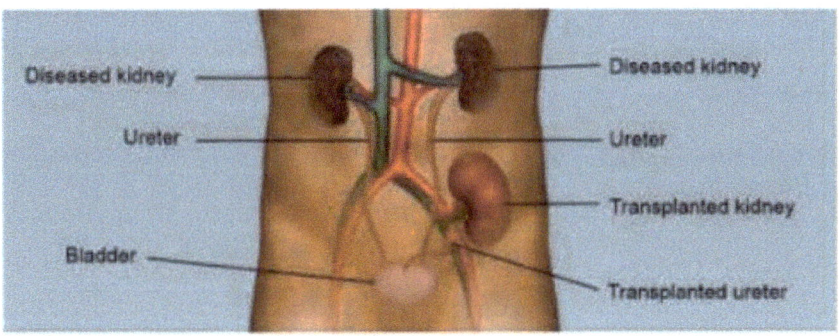

A kidney transplant is performed to place a healthy kidney inside a person who has suffered from kidney failure. The procedure involves surgically placing the donated kidney into the body of an individual whose kidneys have stopped functioning. The kidney can be donated by either a living or deceased donor.

A kidney transplant allows those whose kidneys are no longer functioning to live healthy lives and function more or less like normal individuals. Most importantly, it eliminates the need for lifelong dialysis.

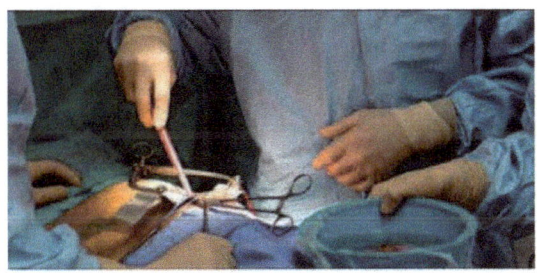

As discussed earlier in the book, the kidneys are two bean-shaped organs located on each side of the spine, roughly the size of a clenched fist, and positioned under the abdomen. Kidneys filter and remove waste, unwanted minerals, and fluids from the bloodstream via urine.

To summarize what was previously studied, when kidneys lose their ability to filter blood, harmful fluids and toxic waste accumulate in the body. This can raise blood pressure and ultimately result in kidney failure, also known as end-stage renal disease (ESRD). ESRD occurs when kidneys lose about 90 percent of their ability to function normally. The buildup of toxins leads to systemic failure, eventually resulting in heart failure and death. Therefore, seeking treatment through alternative methods is vital to sustain life.

Common causes of end-stage kidney disease include:

- Diabetes
- Uncontrolled high blood pressure persisting for long periods
- Chronic glomerulonephritis (inflammation leading to scarring of the tiny filters in the kidneys)
- Polycystic kidney disease

Since it is crucial for patients with ESRD to remove waste products from their bloodstream, dialysis or a kidney transplant becomes imperative for survival. Without one of these treatments, death is inevitable.

Why is a kidney transplant necessary?

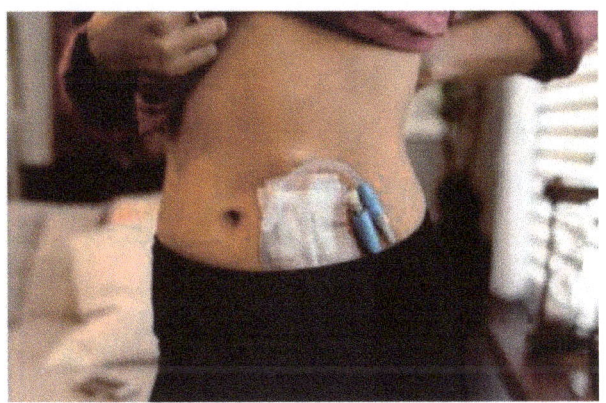

A kidney transplant becomes necessary when the kidneys can no longer perform their essential function of filtering waste and excess fluids from the blood. This condition, known as end-stage renal disease (ESRD) or kidney failure, can result from chronic kidney disease caused by conditions such as diabetes, hypertension, polycystic kidney disease, or glomerulonephritis.

While dialysis can help sustain life by mechanically filtering the blood, it does not replace all kidney functions and often requires strict dietary restrictions and frequent treatments that can significantly affect daily living. In contrast, a kidney transplant provides a more complete and long-term solution by restoring natural kidney function. It allows recipients to lead healthier, more active lives with fewer limitations on diet and fluid intake, improved energy levels, and a reduced risk of complications associated with dialysis.

Moreover, kidney transplantation has been shown to improve life expectancy, enhance fertility, support better cardiovascular health, and contribute to overall mental and emotional well-being, offering a pathway toward a more normal lifestyle for individuals with kidney failure.

Advantages of a kidney transplant include:

- Improved quality of life
- Lower risk of death
- Fewer dietary restrictions
- Lower long-term treatment costs

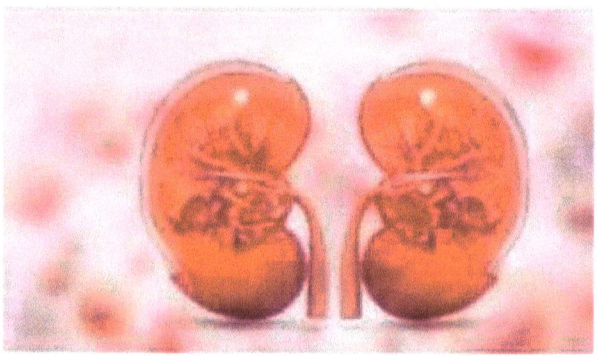

Patients can also benefit from receiving a kidney transplant before they begin dialysis, a procedure known as a preemptive kidney transplant. One of the greatest benefits of transplantation is freedom from lifelong dialysis, allowing recipients to lead more active and fulfilling lives.

Since people can survive with only one functioning kidney, living-donor kidney transplantation is a viable and life-saving option.

Waiting Period for a Donor Kidney

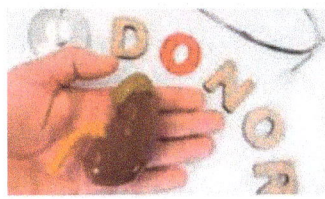

If a compatible living donor is not available, the patient's name is placed on a national or regional kidney transplant waiting list to receive a kidney from a deceased donor. The length of time a patient waits can vary greatly and depends on several key factors:

- **Blood type and tissue compatibility:** A close match between donor and recipient increases the likelihood of a successful transplant.

- **Patient's time on dialysis or on the waitlist:** In many countries, the waiting time is calculated from when the patient started dialysis or was added to the list.

- **Geographic location and organ availability:** Areas with higher organ donation rates may have shorter wait times.

- **Predicted survival benefit:** Some programs prioritize patients who are expected to benefit most from the transplant.

- **Urgency and overall health condition:** Patients with

certain medical needs may be prioritized.

Waiting time can range from a few months to several years. During this period, patients continue regular dialysis and undergo periodic evaluations to ensure they remain healthy enough for surgery when a kidney becomes available.

The kidney transplant procedure

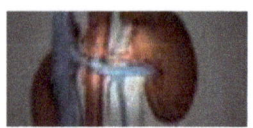

If a living donor is available, the surgery is scheduled in advance. However, if the patient is waiting for a deceased donor, they must be ready to go to the hospital immediately when a kidney becomes available. Transplant centers often provide pagers or cell phones to ensure quick communication when a donor kidney is identified.

Upon arrival at the transplant center, a blood sample is taken to perform an antibody test. If the crossmatch result is negative, clearance for surgery is granted.

The transplant is performed under general anesthesia. The patient is put to sleep using medication administered through an intravenous line in the hand or arm. Once asleep, the surgeon makes an incision in the abdomen and places the donor kidney inside the recipient's body. The donor kidney's arteries and veins are connected to the recipient's blood vessels, allowing blood to flow through the new kidney.

To restore urination, the donor kidney's ureter (the tube connecting the kidney to the bladder) is attached to the recipient's bladder. The original non-functioning kidneys are usually left in place unless they are causing complications such as high blood pressure or infection.

Aftercare Following a Kidney Transplant

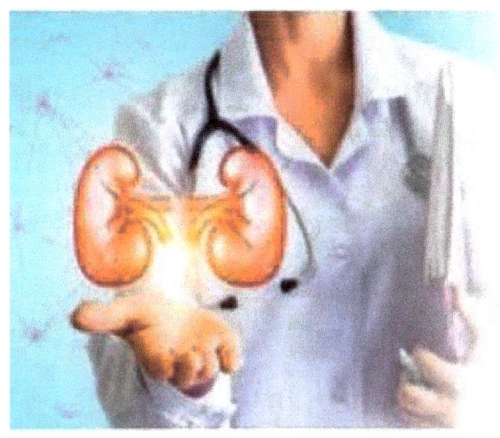

After the transplant surgery is completed, the patient is moved to a recovery room where they are closely monitored as they awaken from anesthesia. Vital signs such as heart rate, blood pressure, and oxygen levels are continuously observed to ensure stability. Once the patient is stable, they are transferred to a specialized hospital room or transplant unit for ongoing care.

The average hospital stay is about one week, even if the patient feels well soon after surgery. This period is crucial for:

- **Monitoring kidney function:** Blood tests are performed frequently to confirm that the transplanted kidney is working properly.

- **Managing fluid and electrolyte balance:** Adjustments are made to prevent dehydration or overload.

- **Detecting early complications:** Such as bleeding, infection, or rejection episodes.

- **Adjusting medications:** Immunosuppressive drugs are started immediately to prevent the immune system from attacking the new kidney. Dosages are carefully tailored to the individual's needs.

- **Education and preparation for discharge:** Patients and caregivers receive guidance on medication schedules, lifestyle changes, signs of rejection, and follow-up appointments.

Even after discharge, close follow-up is required for several months, including frequent lab work and clinic visits to ensure long-term transplant success.

How Quickly Does the New Kidney Start Functioning?

The time it takes for a transplanted kidney to begin working varies widely among recipients and depends on several factors, including the type of donor and the recipient's overall health.

In many cases, especially when the kidney comes from a **living donor**, the new kidney begins filtering blood and producing urine almost immediately after surgery. This is often referred to as **immediate graft function**, and it reduces the need for post-transplant dialysis.

However, in some cases, particularly with **deceased donor kidneys**, there may be a delay known as **delayed graft function (DGF)**. This occurs when the new kidney does not start working right away and may require dialysis for days or even weeks after the transplant. DGF is usually temporary and often resolves as the kidney recovers from the stress of removal, preservation, and transplantation.

Research also shows that kidneys donated by close relatives or genetically similar individuals have a higher chance of working immediately because of better compatibility and reduced risk of immune rejection. Factors like the donor's age, organ quality, preservation time, and the recipient's health can also influence how quickly the kidney starts functioning.

Regular blood tests and urine output monitoring help the transplant team assess kidney function in the critical days following surgery.

What to Expect Following a Kidney Transplant

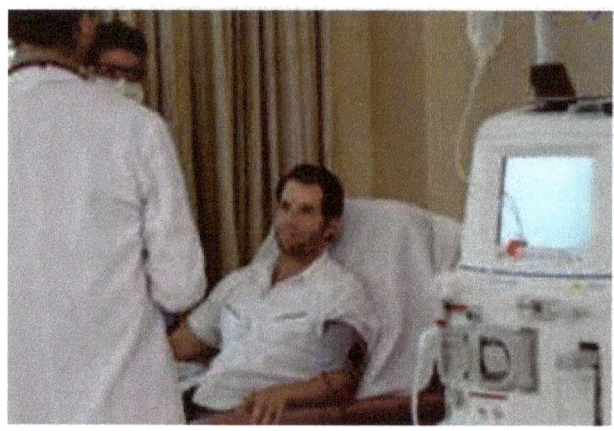

After kidney transplant surgery, recipients can expect a recovery period that involves both physical healing and adjustments to a new medication regimen.

Immediately after the operation, patients often experience **pain, soreness, and swelling** around the incision site. This discomfort is normal and managed with prescribed pain medications. The hospital stay typically lasts about one week, during which doctors closely monitor kidney function, vital signs, and healing progress.

During this time, patients will undergo:

- **Frequent blood tests and urine checks** to assess how well the new kidney is working.
- **Education sessions** on caring for the new kidney, recognizing signs of rejection or infection, and maintaining a healthy lifestyle post-transplant.

- **Physical activity guidance**, as gentle movement is encouraged early to promote circulation and prevent complications like blood clots.

A major part of post-transplant care involves taking **immunosuppressant medications** to prevent the immune system from attacking the new kidney. These drugs must be taken exactly as prescribed for life. Missing doses or stopping them suddenly can result in rejection and potential kidney failure.

Over time, most patients notice improved energy levels, fewer dietary restrictions compared to dialysis, and a significant enhancement in quality of life. However, ongoing follow-up visits are essential to ensure long-term success.

What happens after discharge from the hospital

Most kidney transplant recipients are discharged from the hospital within one to two weeks after surgery. Before leaving, doctors provide detailed instructions regarding medications, follow-up appointments, and lifestyle adjustments. It is critical for the recipient to fully understand these instructions and ask questions about anything unclear. Misunderstanding or missing doses of prescribed medications can lead to organ rejection.

In addition to immunosuppressants, recipients may be given other medications to lower the risk of infection. A schedule for regular checkups is also established. These appointments allow the transplant team to evaluate kidney function and identify any complications early.

Patients must remain vigilant for signs of rejection, which can include:

- Persistent pain or swelling
- Flu-like symptoms such as fever and chills
- Decreased urine output or changes in urination patterns

Recovery from a kidney transplant can take up to six months, with the most critical follow-up period being the first two months after surgery. Consistent communication with the medical team and adherence to all prescribed treatments are essential for a successful recovery.

Benefits of a kidney transplant

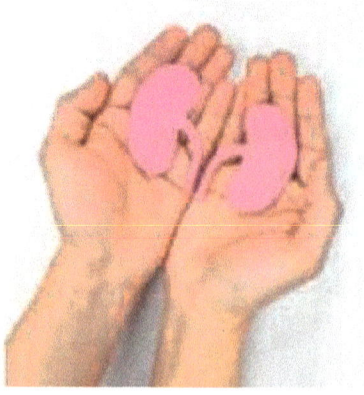

A kidney transplant is widely considered the best treatment option for individuals with long-term kidney disease, offering significant advantages over dialysis.

Key benefits include:

1. No longer needing dialysis

Dialysis is life-saving for people with ESRD but is time-consuming, restrictive, and associated with a high risk of infection. A successful transplant eliminates the need for dialysis, allowing patients to live longer and healthier lives.

2. Increased energy and improved quality of life

Patients who undergo transplantation often report higher energy levels. This improvement allows them to resume daily activities, work, travel, and even exercise or play sports. Compared to dialysis, life after a transplant is generally less restrictive and far more fulfilling.

3. Extended life expectancy

Transplant recipients typically live longer than those who remain on dialysis, as the procedure restores kidney function and reduces complications linked to long-term dialysis dependence.

Reduction in Dietary Restrictions

One of the most noticeable benefits of receiving a kidney transplant is the significant reduction in dietary and fluid limitations. Patients undergoing dialysis must follow very strict guidelines to control

potassium, phosphorus, sodium, and fluid intake because their kidneys are no longer able to remove excess waste and maintain proper electrolyte balance. This often means avoiding many common foods, limiting fruits, dairy, and high-protein meals, and restricting daily fluid consumption to prevent complications such as swelling and heart strain.

After a successful kidney transplant, the new kidney performs these functions more effectively, allowing recipients to **relax many of these restrictions**. While some dietary recommendations remain, such as maintaining a balanced diet, managing weight, and reducing salt to protect kidney health, patients generally enjoy **greater variety and freedom in food choices**. They can also drink fluids more liberally, which contributes to a higher quality of life and makes social activities and daily living more enjoyable.

It is still important for transplant recipients to work with dietitians and follow medical advice, as certain foods may interact with **immunosuppressant medications** or increase infection risk. However, the overall dietary flexibility post-transplant is a major improvement compared to life on dialysis.

Improvement in sex life and fertility

Kidney transplantation can also greatly improve sexual health and fertility compared to patients who remain on dialysis. After a successful transplant, women of childbearing age often regain the ability to conceive.

In some cases, the transplant team may advise a woman to wait for about a year before attempting to conceive to ensure the stability of her health and the transplanted kidney. Overall, sexual function and fertility see a notable improvement following transplantation.

Kidney transplant outlook in the United States

The survival rates for patients diagnosed with long-term kidney disease in the United States have steadily improved over the past three decades. Although there is still room for further improvement, current outcomes are far more promising than in previous years.

Experts and medical professionals strongly support kidney transplantation based on available research and statistics. For most individuals suffering from end-stage kidney disease, transplantation offers a much better quality of life compared to remaining on dialysis indefinitely. While some kidney grafts do fail over time, advances in medical treatment have prolonged the survival of transplanted kidneys, improving patients' overall lifespan and reducing the burden on the healthcare system.

Encouragingly, these advances also increase the availability of kidneys for the approximately 90,000 people currently waiting for a transplant nationwide. Since the mid-1990s, both patient survival rates and graft survival rates have shown steady improvement, even in the face of rising risk factors in the general population such as diabetes, obesity, and related conditions.

Healthcare organizations in the United States have highlighted these positive trends as a sign of continued progress in transplant medicine. This progress underscores the importance of careful donor screening and compatibility testing, along with lifelong use of immunosuppressive drugs to prevent organ rejection.

The five-year survival rate data further illustrates how kidney transplant outcomes have improved in recent decades, offering hope and reassurance to patients awaiting this life-saving procedure.

	Deceased donors	Living donors
1996–1999	66.2%	79.5%
2012–2015	78.2%	88.1%

15: Benefits Of Medicare Coverage for End Stage Renal Disease (ESRD) People

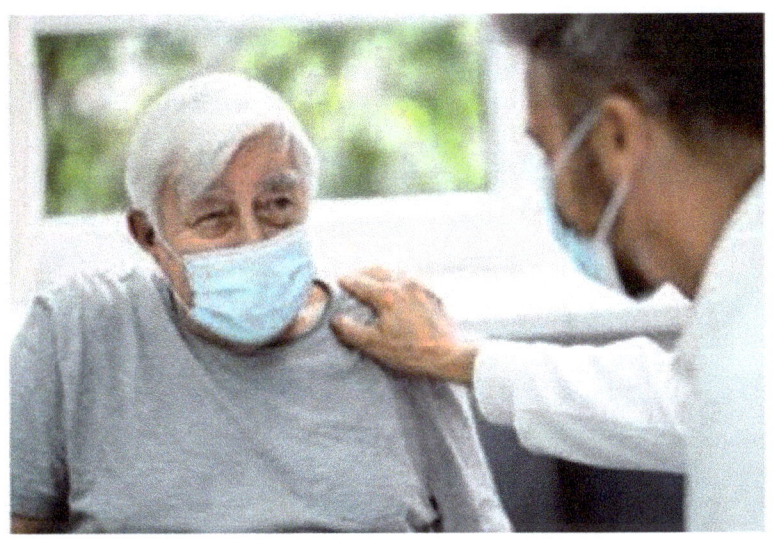

Numerous programs have been aimed at saving and improving the lives of Americans suffering from different ailments, especially at the federal level. However, the Medicare End Stage Renal Disease (ESRD) program, initiated in 1973, stands out as one of the most significant public health initiatives in U.S. history. It has allowed more than one million Americans to benefit from life saving renal replacement therapy, primarily through dialysis and kidney transplantation.

This program marked an unprecedented move, as it became the first federal health insurance program to cover a specific disease rather than an age group or income bracket. Its creation ensured that individuals with ESRD, regardless of age or financial status, could access treatment critical for survival. Without this initiative, most of these individuals would have otherwise died due to the unaffordable cost of care.

The Medicare ESRD program emerged from the Social Security Amendments of 1972, passed by Congress after growing public awareness of the devastating impact of kidney failure. In the early 1970s, the technology for dialysis and kidney transplantation was available but extremely limited. Dialysis machines were scarce, treatments were expensive, and only a select few patients could receive therapy.

Prior to the program's implementation, hospitals and specialized clinics formed "life and death committees," sometimes referred to as "God committees," tasked with deciding which patients would receive dialysis. These decisions were often based on criteria such as age, occupation, family status, and perceived social worth, leaving many to die despite having a treatable condition.

The establishment of Medicare coverage for ESRD fundamentally transformed this landscape. By guaranteeing coverage for dialysis and transplant services, the program not only saved lives but also spurred rapid advancements in nephrology, dialysis technology, and transplant medicine. Over the decades, it has continued to evolve to include home dialysis options, coordinated care models, and incentives for improving patient outcomes and quality of life.

Today, the Medicare ESRD program remains a cornerstone of U.S. healthcare policy, serving as a model for disease specific federal programs and highlighting the role of public health initiatives in addressing chronic, life threatening conditions.

Medicare Coverage for ESRD Patients

The introduction of the Medicare End Stage Renal Disease (ESRD) program brought about a transformative change in healthcare policy and patient outcomes in the United States. Today, every American citizen diagnosed with ESRD is eligible for Medicare benefits, regardless of age. This represents a major departure from traditional Medicare, which generally serves individuals aged 65 and older or those with specific disabilities.

Unlike other federal health programs that impose age or income restrictions, the ESRD program was specifically designed to remove barriers to life saving care for patients facing irreversible kidney failure. Under this program, Medicare provides comprehensive coverage for the medical expenses associated with late stage kidney disease, including dialysis treatments, kidney transplantation, and related services.

ESRD is classified as an advanced chronic condition in which the kidneys have permanently lost their ability to function, making it impossible for the body to filter waste and excess fluids naturally.

Without intervention, this condition is fatal. As a result, patients are left with only two treatment options for survival: long term dialysis, performed either in a clinical setting or at home, or a kidney transplant.

The expansion of Medicare to include ESRD patients regardless of age has provided a critical lifeline to thousands of individuals who, prior to this policy, faced limited treatment options and overwhelming financial burdens. This coverage not only ensures access to essential therapies but also supports broader public health goals by reducing preventable deaths and improving quality of life for those living with chronic kidney failure.

End Stage Renal Disease Treatment Choice (ETC) Model

The End Stage Renal Disease Treatment Choice (ETC) model, introduced and finalized by the Centers for Medicare and Medicaid Services (CMS) in 2020, represents a significant step forward in improving access to care for patients diagnosed with ESRD. This model was designed to address long-standing gaps in coverage and ensure that patients could receive life saving treatments without the financial and administrative burdens previously associated with chronic kidney disease care.

Before the implementation of the ETC model, many patients faced challenges such as loss of coverage, higher insurance premiums, and limited options for dialysis or transplant services. By creating a standardized approach, the ETC model has helped protect ESRD patients from losing health coverage or being overcharged, ultimately making essential therapies like dialysis and transplantation more accessible.

The model also incentivizes better quality of care and encourages providers to offer home dialysis options when clinically appropriate. This focus on coordinated and patient-centered care reflects broader reforms in Medicare aimed at improving outcomes while managing costs.

ESRD Patients with Private Insurance and Group Coverage

For patients who have private insurance or are covered by an employer-sponsored group health plan, the ETC model establishes important protections. Group health plan providers are expressly forbidden from discriminating against ESRD patients by limiting benefits, terminating coverage, or increasing premiums solely due to the ESRD diagnosis. These provisions ensure that individuals are not financially penalized for their condition.

Patients with group health plan coverage must enroll in Medicare within 30 months following an ESRD diagnosis. This 30-month period is known as the **coordination period**.

During this coordination period:

- The **group health insurance** serves as the **primary payer**, covering most healthcare costs related to ESRD treatment.

- **Medicare** functions as the **secondary payer**, covering any remaining approved expenses.

After the 30-month coordination period ends, this arrangement reverses: Medicare becomes the primary payer, while the group health plan assumes secondary coverage.

Enrollment in Medicare and the timing of coverage can vary depending on whether the patient receives dialysis treatments or undergoes a kidney transplant. Understanding this timeline is crucial for patients and families planning long-term care and financial arrangements.

Dialysis Treatment and Medicare

For ESRD patients treated with dialysis, Medicare benefits begin in the fourth month of treatment. Dialysis must be received in a Medicare approved dialysis center.

However, if ESRD patients learn to administer dialysis at home, they may be eligible for Medicare benefits earlier. In some cases, treatment costs may be covered from the first month of dialysis if:

- The patient undergoes and completes a training program from a Medicare approved facility for home dialysis.

- The patient begins a home dialysis training program

- The patient performs self dialysis during the first three months.

ESRD patients receiving dialysis will continue to receive Medicare benefits for 12 months following the last month of dialysis treatment.

Kidney Transplant and Medicare

Kidney transplantation is often considered the most effective long-term treatment for patients with End Stage Renal Disease (ESRD). Under Medicare, individuals admitted to a Medicare-approved facility or hospital for a kidney transplant, or any preparatory transplant-related services required within two months, become eligible to receive Medicare benefits during that same month.

This coverage includes the surgery itself, pre-transplant evaluations, hospital stays, and immediate post-operative care. In addition, Medicare often covers follow-up appointments, lab tests, and medications necessary for the stabilization of the new kidney during the initial recovery phase.

Transplant recipients can continue benefiting from Medicare for up to 36 months after the transplant procedure. If a patient's kidney transplant fails and they require either renewed dialysis or a second transplant, they may again qualify for coverage under the End Stage

Renal Disease Treatment Choice (ETC) model. In such situations, the 30-month coordination period between private insurance and Medicare applies once more, ensuring patients are not left without coverage during critical transitions in care.

Services Covered by Medicare

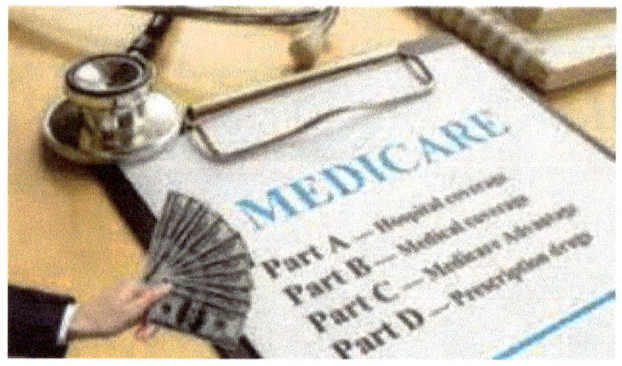

While most individuals associate ESRD coverage with dialysis and kidney transplantation, Medicare also provides a broader range of medical services necessary to treat related complications and maintain overall health. These include:

- **Inpatient hospital care** related to ESRD complications or treatment.

- **Outpatient services**, such as lab tests, imaging, and follow-up care connected to kidney disease management.

- **Home health services**, particularly for patients undergoing home dialysis.

- **Preventive care** to monitor and manage comorbid conditions, including diabetes and hypertension, which frequently accompany ESRD.

It is important to note that Medicare only pays for services it approves. Prescription drugs, including post-transplant immunosuppressive medications, are not covered under standard Medicare Parts A and B. To access prescription drug coverage, ESRD patients must enroll in an additional plan, such as:

- A standalone Medicare Part D prescription drug plan.
- A Medicare Advantage plan with integrated drug coverage.
- Creditable prescription coverage through an employer or union plan.

Without this supplemental coverage, patients could face substantial out-of-pocket expenses for critical medications.

Medicare's Special Plans

Because ESRD is a highly complex condition requiring intensive and coordinated care, Medicare has developed specialized options to meet these patients' unique needs. **Medicare Advantage Special Needs Plans (SNPs)** are designed specifically for individuals with chronic conditions like ESRD.

These plans combine the hospital and medical coverage of Medicare Parts A and B, often include prescription drug coverage (Part D), and may provide additional benefits that traditional Medicare does not, such as:

- Dental, vision, and hearing services.
- Transportation to dialysis centers or transplant follow-up appointments.
- Care coordination programs to help manage multiple specialists and treatments.
- Nutrition counseling and other supportive services aimed at improving quality of life.

These targeted benefits make Medicare Advantage Special Needs Plans a valuable resource for patients managing ESRD, offering comprehensive support that addresses both medical and non-medical challenges associated with the condition.

Conditions for Coverage Ending, Continuing, or Resuming

Medicare coverage will end for individuals who qualify solely due to ESRD:

- Twelve months after stopping dialysis, or
- Thirty six months after receiving a kidney transplant, provided no further dialysis is required.

Coverage will resume if dialysis is restarted within 12 months of stopping treatment or if another kidney transplant occurs within 36 months. Patients who resume dialysis or undergo another transplant within this period will continue receiving Medicare benefits.

The Medicare coverage for patients with ESRD will resume if it ends and the patient restarts dialysis or undergoes another kidney transplant for kidney failure. In such cases, the Medicare coverage will start immediately without any waiting period.

Eligibility Criteria for Medicare if a Patient Has ESRD

If an individual has been diagnosed with ESRD, Medicare can be received regardless of age under the following conditions:

- The individual's kidneys no longer work.
- The individual requires regular dialysis.
- The individual has received a kidney transplant.
- The individual has fulfilled the required amount of time under Social Security, as a government employee, or under the Railroad Retirement Board (RRB).
- Individuals who are already availing or are eligible for Social Security or Railroad Retirement benefits.
- The individual is a spouse or dependent of a person who fulfills the above conditions.

ESRD Patients and Medicare Advantage

Medicare Advantage

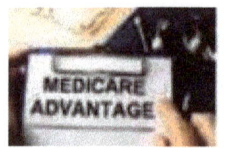 Medicare Advantage, or MA, is an option for individuals on Medicare coverage diagnosed with ESRD. Medicare Advantage is also called Medicare Part C. It is a comprehensive program that functions as an all-in-one health insurance plan. It combines the benefits of Medicare Parts A, B, and sometimes Part D, making it a convenient option.

Benefits of Medicare Advantage for ESRD Patients

There are numerous benefits to choosing Medicare Advantage:

1. ESRD patients will only need to manage one plan for all their healthcare needs, meaning only one insurance card is required.

2. Some plans may have costs equal to or lower than traditional Medicare, with premiums sometimes as low as 0 dollars.

3. Many plans include additional benefits, such as dental, vision, and hearing care.

4. Patients can save on prescription costs, including kidney medications and insulin.

5. Spending is capped due to annual out-of-pocket cost limits.

Medicare Advantage Compared to Other Medicare Plans

Medicare Advantage replaces Medicare Parts A and B and often includes Part D. Comparing the costs, benefits, and potential savings makes this plan a strong choice for those diagnosed with ESRD.

When an ESRD patient selects a Medicare Advantage plan with prescription coverage, the patient is fully insured under one plan. This eliminates the need for a separate prescription plan with its own premium. This integration helps individuals save money while enjoying comprehensive health coverage.

Medicare Advantage also offers additional benefits not available under traditional Medicare, including dental, vision, hearing care, and transportation services.

A key difference is that Medicare Advantage plans are managed by private health insurance companies, whereas traditional Medicare is managed by the federal government.

Choosing Between Medicare Advantage and Traditional Medicare

One of the key decisions facing patients diagnosed with End Stage Renal Disease (ESRD) is whether to enroll in **Medicare Advantage (Part C)** or remain with **Traditional Medicare (Parts A and B)**. Both options provide coverage for essential treatments such as dialysis and kidney transplantation, but they differ in structure, costs, and additional benefits.

A major advantage of Medicare Advantage plans is their use of **provider networks**, often similar to employer-sponsored group health plans. This network model allows individuals to choose in-network doctors and facilities, which helps reduce out-of-pocket expenses and streamline care coordination. In addition, Medicare Advantage plans frequently bundle services, hospital care, outpatient care, and prescription drug coverage, into a single comprehensive plan, eliminating the need for multiple separate enrollments.

By comparison, Traditional Medicare typically requires patients to combine different parts (A, B, and optionally D) and may leave gaps in coverage that must be filled with **Medigap supplemental insurance**. For ESRD patients seeking simplicity and predictable costs, Medicare Advantage can be especially appealing.

In summary, Medicare Advantage offers:

- Lower or capped out-of-pocket costs in many plans.
- A single insurance card covering hospital, outpatient, and often prescription benefits.
- Additional perks, such as dental, vision, and transportation benefits, not typically available under Traditional Medicare.

While Medicare Advantage provides convenience and potentially lower costs, patients must still consider factors like provider network restrictions, regional plan availability, and individual healthcare needs. Carefully reviewing plan details remains essential before making a decision.

Supplemental Insurance and Medicare Advantage

Patients enrolled in Medicare Advantage plans generally do **not** require supplemental insurance. This is because Medicare Advantage plans are designed as an all-in-one alternative to Traditional Medicare, often including prescription drug coverage (Part D) and other benefits in the same package.

Since all coverage is consolidated into a single plan:

- There is **no need to purchase a separate prescription drug plan**.
- There is **no need for a Medicare Supplement (Medigap) policy**.
- Patients can manage all their healthcare needs through one insurance provider, simplifying billing, paperwork, and access to services.

This streamlined approach can be particularly valuable for ESRD patients, who often require ongoing, coordinated care and frequent medical appointments. By reducing the need to manage multiple insurance plans, Medicare Advantage allows patients to focus more on treatment and recovery rather than navigating complex administrative tasks.

16: Healthy Lifestyle

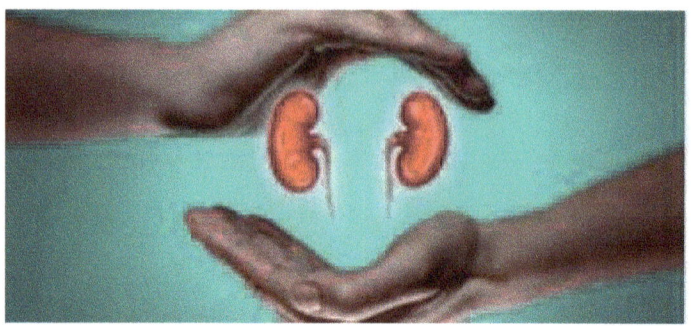

The kidneys are important organs about the size of a fist, located at the bottom of the rib cage. Found on both sides of the spine, the kidneys perform several essential functions critical to sustaining life. Among their many vital roles, they filter the bloodstream by eliminating excess water, waste products, and other impurities via urine through the bladder.

In addition to this crucial function, the kidneys regulate pH, salt, and potassium levels, helping maintain the body's delicate chemical balance. They also play a key role in regulating blood pressure by secreting the hormone renin, which influences the constriction of blood vessels and fluid balance in the body. Furthermore, the kidneys produce erythropoietin, a hormone that stimulates the production of red blood cells in the bone marrow, ensuring that tissues receive adequate oxygen.

The kidneys have other important roles as well. They activate a form of vitamin D called calcitriol, which is necessary to help the body absorb calcium and phosphorus from the diet. This is essential not only for building strong bones but also for regulating muscle function and supporting a healthy immune system.

Structurally, each kidney contains around one million tiny filtering units called nephrons. These nephrons filter the blood, selectively reabsorb needed substances, and excrete waste as urine. The kidneys receive about 20 to 25 percent of the heart's blood output, emphasizing their importance in overall circulation and detoxification.

Because of the many important functions of the kidneys, it is imperative to maintain kidney health. This is critical to your overall well-being. Healthy kidneys help the body filter and expel waste adequately. Without removing these waste products, toxins can build up in the body, leading to serious health problems such as kidney failure or systemic complications.

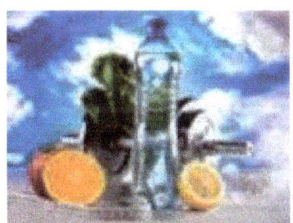

Additionally, the hormones required to help the body function properly will only be produced with healthy kidneys. Kidney disease or damage can disrupt these functions, causing imbalances in electrolytes, blood pressure, and red blood cell levels. To support kidney health, it is important to stay hydrated, eat a balanced diet low in excessive salt and processed foods, manage blood sugar and blood pressure, and avoid excessive use of medications that can harm the kidneys.

Early detection and management of kidney problems through regular medical check-ups can prevent the progression of kidney disease, helping maintain a good quality of life.

Importance of Preventing Chronic Kidney Disease and the Risk Factors

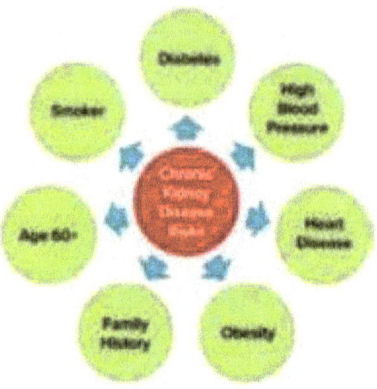

Many risk factors increase the chances of developing chronic kidney disease (CKD). Individuals with certain underlying health conditions are more likely to experience kidney problems. The most common risk factors include:

- Diabetes
- High blood pressure
- Heart disease
- Family history of kidney failure

Uncovering the Root Causes of Dialysis Needs

If you have any of these conditions, your risk of developing kidney disease is considerably higher. This is because conditions like diabetes and high blood pressure can damage the small blood vessels in the kidneys, impairing their ability to filter blood effectively over time.

Fortunately, the health of your kidneys can be maintained, and further damage can often be prevented by managing and controlling these underlying health issues. Effective treatment and lifestyle changes aimed at keeping blood sugar and blood pressure within healthy ranges play a crucial role in protecting your kidneys.

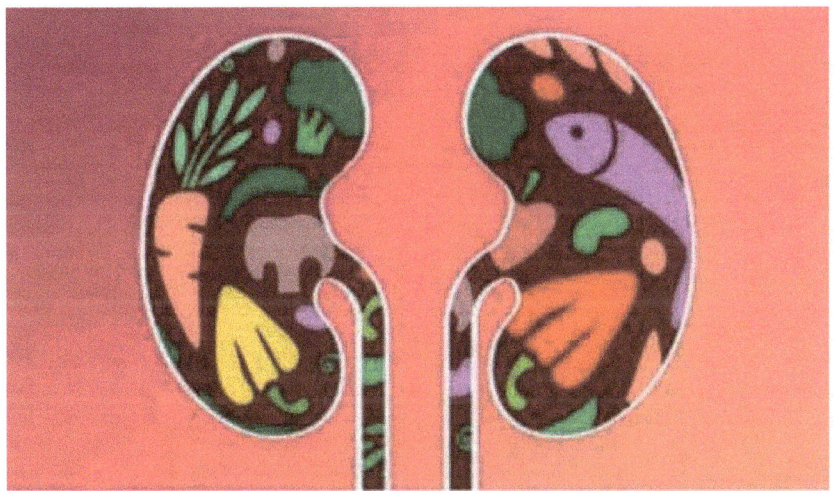

Here are some important steps you can take to ensure your kidneys — and your entire body — remain healthy and function optimally:

- Maintain a balanced diet low in salt, processed foods, and excessive sugars

- Stay adequately hydrated by drinking plenty of water
- Exercise regularly to support cardiovascular health
- Avoid smoking and limit alcohol consumption
- Follow your healthcare provider's recommendations for managing chronic conditions

Regular monitoring of your kidney health is essential because kidney disease often develops silently without noticeable symptoms in the early stages. The only way to detect early kidney damage is through specific medical tests. Whenever you go for a medical checkup, make sure to ask your healthcare provider to evaluate your kidney function. Common tests include blood tests to measure creatinine and calculate estimated glomerular filtration rate (eGFR), as well as urine tests to check for protein or blood.

Based on the test results, your doctor can determine how frequently you should be tested to keep a close watch on your kidney health. Early detection allows timely intervention, preventing problems from escalating and reducing the risk of kidney failure.

In addition to chronic conditions, kidney damage can also result from infections such as urinary tract infections (UTIs). These infections, if left untreated, can spread to the kidneys and cause serious damage. A kidney function test can help identify such infections early so that they can be promptly treated to avoid complications.

By understanding your risk factors, proactively monitoring your kidney health, and adopting a healthy lifestyle, you can significantly reduce your chances of developing chronic kidney disease and maintain overall well-being.

Healthy Food Intake

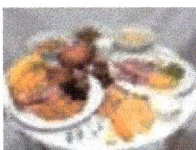
Selecting the right foods to eat is very important for maintaining overall health, including the health of your kidneys and heart. Following a proper, balanced diet can help improve and sustain your body's vital functions.

To support kidney health, focus on choosing foods that are nutritious and low in harmful substances. Fresh fruits and vegetables are excellent choices because they provide essential vitamins, minerals, and antioxidants that help reduce inflammation and promote healthy organ function.

Incorporating whole grains such as brown rice, quinoa, oats, and whole wheat products into your meals provides fiber and important nutrients that support digestion and cardiovascular health. Pairing these with low-fat or fat-free dairy products can further help maintain healthy bones and provide protein without excess unhealthy fats.

It is important to limit your intake of salt (sodium) and added sugars, as excessive amounts can strain your kidneys and increase the risk of high blood pressure and other health problems. The recommended daily sodium intake is less than 2,300 milligrams—about one teaspoon of salt. Reducing sodium helps control blood pressure and decreases the workload on your kidneys.

Similarly, try to limit added sugars to less than 10 percent of your daily calorie intake. Excess sugars can contribute to weight gain, diabetes, and inflammation, all of which negatively impact kidney function.

Other dietary tips for kidney health include:

- Choosing lean proteins such as fish, poultry, and plant-based proteins like beans and lentils, which put less strain on the kidneys compared to high-fat meats
- Avoiding processed and packaged foods that often contain hidden sodium and unhealthy fats
- Drinking plenty of water to help flush waste from the kidneys and keep the body hydrated

By following these dietary guidelines, you can help protect your kidneys, support heart health, and promote overall well-being.

How to Make Healthy Food Choices

Uncovering the Root Causes of Dialysis Needs

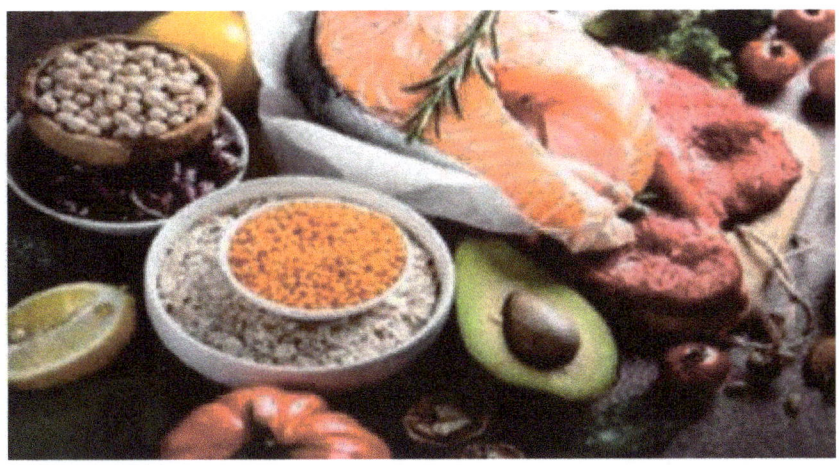

There are many useful tips for making healthy food choices that can help protect your kidneys and improve your overall well-being. One simple change is to cook with a mix of herbs and spices instead of relying on salt to flavor your meals. Spices like garlic, ginger, turmeric, and black pepper not only add delicious taste but also provide health benefits. For example, choosing vegetable toppings like broccoli on your dishes or peppers on pizza adds important nutrients and fiber that support your health.

When it comes to cooking methods, opt for baking, steaming, boiling, or grilling rather than frying. Fried foods tend to be high in unhealthy fats that can contribute to kidney strain and heart disease. Boiling meat, chicken, or fish without adding heavy sauces or gravies is a healthier choice that reduces excess fat and calories. Avoid foods with gravy and added fats, and steer clear of added sugars as much as possible. Always select foods that contain little or no added sugar to maintain a healthy diet.

Dairy products can also impact kidney and heart health. It is helpful to reduce whole milk intake and replace it with lower-fat options such as 2 percent milk or fat-free (skim) milk. Low-fat milk and milk products provide the necessary calcium and protein without excessive saturated fat.

Incorporating whole grains into your daily diet is another essential step. Whole grains such as whole wheat, brown rice, oats, and whole-grain corn provide fiber, vitamins, and minerals that support digestion and cardiovascular health. Use whole-grain bread for toast and sandwiches and substitute brown rice for white rice, both at home and when eating out. These small swaps contribute significantly to a healthier eating pattern.

Reading food labels carefully before purchasing products helps you make informed choices. Pay attention to the amounts of saturated fats, trans fats, sodium (salt), added sugars, and cholesterol. Choosing foods low in these ingredients can help reduce your risk of kidney problems and maintain your overall health.

Another important habit is managing snacking behaviors. Try to reduce consumption of high-calorie snacks and replace them with lower-calorie alternatives. For example, eating a bag of low-fat popcorn is a better option than cake or other sugary snacks. Instead of drinking orange juice, peel and eat an orange to benefit from the fiber and reduce calorie intake. These small changes can add up to significant calorie reduction over time.

Keeping a written record of your daily food intake is a helpful practice to avoid overeating or consuming foods high in fat and calories. Tracking your meals can increase awareness of your eating habits and motivate you to make healthier choices.

Research has shown that following a diet based on healthy foods like those mentioned above helps maintain normal blood pressure levels. If you already have high blood pressure, diabetes, heart disease, or other conditions that increase your risk for kidney disease, it is important to consult a dietitian or healthcare professional. They can help design a personalized diet plan tailored to your needs.

Finally, regular physical activity should be an integral part of your lifestyle. Exercise helps control weight, improve blood pressure, and enhance overall kidney and cardiovascular health. Combining a healthy diet with consistent exercise is one of the best ways to protect your kidneys and promote long-term wellness.

Try being active for at least 30 minutes or more each day. If you do not currently engage in activities that require physical exertion, consult with a healthcare provider about how to adapt to an active lifestyle. This will help you determine suitable physical activities to boost your overall health. Guidance from a professional will help you establish a physically active schedule that benefits your well-being.

Always Maintain a Healthy Weight

Maintaining a healthy weight is crucial for your overall health and the well-being of your kidneys. Excess weight or obesity increases the risk of numerous health problems, including kidney damage. If you are overweight or obese, it is important to begin working toward weight loss as soon as possible.

Collaborating with a healthcare provider or registered dietitian can help you develop a realistic, personalized weight-loss plan. These professionals can guide you in making sustainable lifestyle changes, focusing on balanced nutrition and increased physical activity. Utilizing available resources for weight management and exercise will support your efforts to lose weight safely and maintain a healthy body weight over time.

Getting enough sleep is another vital component of good health. Experts recommend aiming for 7 to 8 hours of quality, uninterrupted sleep each night. Adequate sleep helps lower stress hormones, supports immune function, and keeps you feeling refreshed and energized throughout the day. If you struggle with sleep, consider adopting healthy sleep habits or consulting a healthcare professional to improve your sleep quality.

Quit smoking if you currently use tobacco in any form. Smoking

Uncovering the Root Causes of Dialysis Needs

causes widespread damage to your health, including reducing blood flow to the kidneys and increasing the risk of kidney disease. If you find it difficult to quit, seek professional support such as counseling or smoking cessation programs.

Limit alcohol intake because excessive drinking can raise blood pressure and add unnecessary calories that contribute to weight gain. Reducing alcohol consumption can help protect your kidneys and improve overall health. Aim to drink in moderation or abstain altogether.

Engage in stress-reducing activities to support both your emotional and physical well-being. Chronic stress negatively affects many body systems, including the kidneys. Consider practices recommended by healthcare professionals such as mindfulness meditation, yoga, deep breathing exercises, or regular physical activity to manage stress effectively.

Finally, **managing key risk factors** such as diabetes, high blood pressure, and heart disease is essential for kidney health. These conditions are among the leading causes of kidney damage worldwide. Keeping them well-controlled through medication, lifestyle changes, and regular medical checkups is the best way to protect your kidneys from long-term harm.

By addressing these factors—healthy weight, sufficient sleep, quitting smoking, moderating alcohol intake, managing stress, and controlling chronic health conditions—you can significantly improve your kidney health and overall quality of life.

Start by keeping your blood glucose levels within a healthy range. Monitoring your blood glucose, also called blood sugar, is crucial in managing diabetes. Your doctor may recommend testing your blood glucose levels multiple times a day.

Maintaining normal blood pressure is also important. For people with diabetes, blood pressure should be below 140/90 mm Hg. If you have high blood pressure, consult your doctor. You may need to adjust your diet or take medications to keep it under control. It is important to take all medicines as prescribed.

You can also discuss with your doctor about certain blood pressure medications, such as ACE inhibitors and ARBs, which can help protect your kidneys.

Be cautious about the daily use of over-the-counter pain medications. Regular use of nonsteroidal anti-inflammatory drugs (NSAIDs), such as ibuprofen, can cause damage to your kidneys and overall health.

You also need to reduce your risk of heart attacks and strokes by keeping cholesterol levels in check. There are two types of cholesterol in your blood: LDL and HDL. LDL is known as "bad" cholesterol because it can build up in your bloodstream and clog blood vessels, leading to heart attacks or strokes. HDL is called

Uncovering the Root Causes of Dialysis Needs

"good" cholesterol because it helps remove LDL from the bloodstream.

You may need to undergo a cholesterol test, which also measures triglycerides, another type of blood fat.

The Important Tasks of Healthy Kidneys at a Glance:

- Regulating the fluid levels in your body
- Filtering wastes and toxins from the bloodstream
- Releasing a hormone responsible for regulating blood pressure
- Activating vitamin D to maintain healthy bones
- Releasing a hormone involved in the production of red blood cells
- Keeping blood minerals in balance, such as sodium, phosphorus, and potassium

Examples of Problems Caused by Kidney Disease:

- Heart disease
- Stroke
- Heart attack
- High blood pressure
- Weak bones

- Nerve damage (neuropathy)
- Kidney failure
- End-stage kidney disease (ESRD)
- Anemia or low red blood cell count

Assessing Your Risk for Kidney Disease

There are five main risk factors that significantly increase your likelihood of developing kidney disease. Controlling these risk factors can help reduce your chances of kidney damage. These include:

- Diabetes
- High blood pressure
- Heart disease
- Family history of kidney failure or any of the conditions mentioned above
- Obesity

In addition to these major risk factors, there are other important conditions and circumstances that can also increase your risk. These additional factors include:

- Being aged 60 or above
- Low birth weight

Uncovering the Root Causes of Dialysis Needs

- Prolonged use of nonsteroidal anti-inflammatory drugs (NSAIDs), such as ibuprofen and naproxen
- Autoimmune diseases like lupus
- Chronic urinary tract infections
- Kidney stones

Why Knowing Your Risk Factors Matters

Understanding and learning about these risk factors increases your awareness of kidney health and allows you to take proactive steps. This knowledge empowers you to make lifestyle choices and seek medical advice that can protect your kidneys, prevent disease progression, and help you lead a healthier life.

Recognizing the symptoms of kidney problems

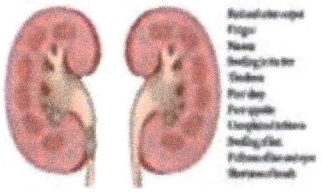

Many signs may suggest trouble. However, most people with early kidney disease show no symptoms. Detecting early symptoms is critical because the disease may be advanced once symptoms appear. Pay close attention to these symptoms:

- Fatigue
- Weakness
- Difficulty urinating
- Blood in urine, with urine turning pink or dark
- Foamy urine
- Increased need to urinate, especially at night
- Increased thirst
- Puffy eyes
- Swelling in the face, hands, or abdomen

Getting tested is important — here is how

If you or a loved one are at high risk for kidney disease, discuss this immediately with a primary care physician, including tests needed to assess risk. Your doctor may order additional tests to evaluate kidney health and damage.

Three Life-Saving Tests to Monitor Kidney Health

1. Blood Pressure Test

High blood pressure (hypertension) damages the tiny blood vessels in the kidneys called glomeruli, which are the key filtering units. This damage impairs kidney function and is the second leading cause of kidney failure after diabetes. Keeping blood pressure under control is essential for protecting your kidneys.

- A blood pressure reading of **140/90 mm Hg** is generally acceptable for most people.
- For individuals with chronic kidney disease (CKD), maintaining blood pressure **below 130/80 mm Hg** is recommended.
- An ideal target is **below 120/80 mm Hg**, but it's important to discuss your personal goals with your doctor.

Regular monitoring helps catch high blood pressure early and enables timely management.

2. Urine Test

A urine test can detect the presence of a protein called **albumin** in your urine, which may be an early sign of kidney disease. Normally, protein should not be found in significant amounts in the urine.

- When albumin is present in small amounts, this condition is called **albuminuria**.
- Higher levels of protein in urine, known as **proteinuria**, indicate more significant kidney damage.

Results showing less than **30 mg of albumin per gram of urinary creatinine** are considered normal. Creatinine is a waste product produced by muscles and filtered by the kidneys. This test helps identify kidney problems before symptoms appear.

3. Glomerular Filtration Rate (GFR)

GFR measures how well your kidneys are filtering blood by estimating how much blood passes through the glomeruli each minute. It is calculated using your blood creatinine levels, age, sex, and other factors.

- A **GFR above 90** is considered normal kidney function.
- A GFR between **60 and 89** requires regular monitoring, especially if other signs of kidney damage exist.
- A sustained GFR **below 60 for three months or more** indicates chronic kidney disease.

Early detection through GFR testing can prevent progression and allow timely intervention.

Staying Healthy with Kidney Disease

If you have been diagnosed with kidney disease, following these guidelines can help slow its progression and maintain your health:

- Maintain blood pressure within your target range
- Control blood sugar levels if you have diabetes
- Avoid nonsteroidal anti-inflammatory drugs (NSAIDs) like ibuprofen and naproxen, which can harm kidneys
- Reduce salt intake to help control blood pressure and fluid balance

Uncovering the Root Causes of Dialysis Needs

- Keep protein consumption moderate to reduce kidney workload
- Get an annual flu shot to prevent infections that can worsen kidney problems

Important Steps to Maintain Good Kidney Health

To protect your kidneys and overall health, consider adopting these healthy habits:

- Exercise regularly to support cardiovascular and kidney health
- Control your weight through balanced nutrition and physical activity
- Follow a diet rich in fresh fruits, vegetables, whole grains, and low in sodium and unhealthy fats
- Quit smoking and limit alcohol consumption
- Stay well hydrated by drinking adequate water daily
- Monitor cholesterol levels and manage any abnormalities
- Attend annual physical checkups, including kidney function tests when recommended
- Learn and understand your family medical history to identify inherited risks

Important Fact about Kidney Disease in the U.S.

Dialysis Champions

Approximately **1 in 10 Americans aged 20 or older** show evidence of kidney disease. Many forms of kidney disease common in the U.S. are progressive, meaning they worsen over time. Eventually, the kidneys may fail and lose their ability to remove waste from the bloodstream. Early detection and management are crucial to preventing kidney failure and maintaining a good quality of life.

17: HOW TO BECOME AN EFFECTIVE NURSE

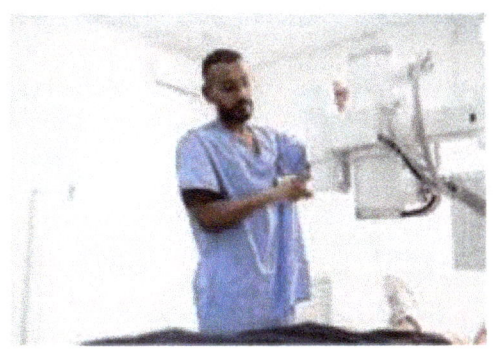

Nurses play a vital role in any healthcare system. Being an effective nurse requires much more than just a degree. As one of the most challenging professional careers, nursing demands many skills to be successful. It is not just a straightforward career path. The role of nursing envisions much more than a high level of education. It mandates a strong sense of dedication to fulfill key responsibilities. Furthermore, physical and mental endurance must be effective in a nursing job. The world outside nursing school is vast, and nurses must equip themselves with specific personality traits and skill sets to improve patients' health outcomes.

To be influential nurses, in addition to top skills, nurses need to be resilient against stress. Here are some qualities that good nurses must embody.

Good organizational behavior is key to the successful dispensation of nursing responsibilities. Experts often cite organization as the essential trait a nurse must demonstrate through their behavior. The medical field has many ups and downs. From a chaotic shift to a patient's health spiraling out of control, nurses must be organized to adapt to challenging times and prioritize what is best for patients.

Nurses have many vital roles to play, and organization becomes a critical skill they must master to make their job easier and positively impact patients and the entire healthcare team. The importance of this trait cannot be underestimated because it is critical to keeping patients safe and ensuring they are healing. Besides, organizational skills are required to keep a close eye on everything happening with patients.

In addition to organization, effective communication skills are fundamental for nursing success. Nurses serve as the primary link between patients, families, and the broader medical team. They must be able to convey complex medical information clearly and compassionately while also listening attentively to patient concerns. This two-way communication helps build trust, reduces patient anxiety, and facilitates collaborative decision-making that enhances care quality.

Compassion and empathy form the emotional backbone of nursing. The ability to connect with patients on a human level, to understand their fears and pain, and to provide comfort is what transforms nursing from a job into a vocation. Nurses who demonstrate genuine care often improve patient satisfaction and promote quicker recovery by fostering a positive healing environment.

Moreover, critical thinking and problem-solving skills are essential in the fast-paced, unpredictable world of healthcare. Nurses frequently encounter situations where quick decisions can significantly impact patient outcomes. They must analyze symptoms, anticipate complications, and collaborate with doctors to adjust treatment plans dynamically. This level of cognitive agility ensures patient safety and effective treatment.

Physical stamina and mental toughness also cannot be overlooked. Nursing shifts can be long and physically demanding, requiring nurses to remain alert and effective throughout. Mental endurance helps them cope with emotionally draining situations, including witnessing suffering and loss, without compromising the quality of care.

Finally, lifelong learning is a hallmark of exemplary nursing professionals. Healthcare is an ever-evolving field with continuous advancements in medical technology, treatment protocols, and patient care strategies. Nurses committed to ongoing education not only maintain their competence but also drive improvements in healthcare delivery.

Being able to multitask and stay organized is essential to be a practical nurse. From noticing small and minor details about the patient to collecting labs and ensuring patients take medications on time, all tasks regarding a patient's health need to be prioritized and organized.

Critical thinking is essential to come up with effective solutions to healthcare challenges. Once again, this is another important skill required to be effective in a healthcare setting. The ability to think logically, clearly, and intellectually is key to successfully fulfilling the responsibilities and tasks assigned to a nurse. This is also one of the nurses' highly demanded skills because, just like good organization, it is critical to ensuring improved patient outcomes. Since it directly impacts patient care and affects health outcomes, critical thinking is essential for offering self-sufficiency to nurses.

Critical thinking is a vital trait that equips nurses with the ability to logically and objectively analyze facts and challenges to find lasting and effective solutions. Without strong critical thinking skills, nurses may struggle to reach sound conclusions, leading to poor decision-making that can adversely affect patient care and their professional growth. This deficiency can result in repeated struggles and setbacks throughout their careers.

To illustrate the importance of critical thinking, consider the case of forensic nursing. This specialized field, by all standards, is both highly rewarding and lucrative but also comes with numerous complex challenges. Nurses in this role must possess a keen eye for detail, combined with deep insight into rational and analytical thinking. Their effectiveness hinges on their ability to participate meticulously in evidence-gathering procedures during investigations of crimes or trauma. Failure to apply critical thinking skills in this context would not only jeopardize the integrity of evidence but could also lead to miscarriages of justice.

Forensic nurses must be adept at interpreting, evaluating, and analyzing facts accurately to contribute meaningfully to legal and medical processes. The same requirement for critical thinking applies broadly across various nursing specialties, from intensive care units to community health settings. Nurses are constantly faced with dynamic, often high-pressure situations that demand swift yet sound judgments. Consequently, critical thinking is not a one-time skill but a continuous learning process that nurses must cultivate throughout their careers.

Good communication skills are equally critical to improving healthcare outcomes. Among the myriad skills nurses need, effective communication stands out as perhaps the most indispensable. Without it, nurses would struggle to fulfill their roles efficiently. Communication goes beyond merely exchanging information; it involves active listening, clear articulation, empathy, and the ability to educate patients and families about care plans, medications, and treatments.

Poor communication can lead to misunderstandings, medication errors, and decreased patient compliance, all of which can jeopardize patient safety. In contrast, nurses who communicate effectively foster trust, reduce anxiety, and improve collaboration within the healthcare team. This collaborative spirit is essential for ensuring that patient care is coordinated and comprehensive.

The role of a nurse requires them to handle much data that needs to be collected and conveyed to the relevant healthcare providers. There is no room for errors in the collection and handling of essential patient data. The data needs to be interpreted as accurately as possible.

Just imagine a scenario where a nurse misses patient information or hears the wrong orders. Consider the consequences of any misinformation from the nurse. All these mistakes endanger the patient's life. A nurse needs to take instructions from coworkers and supervisors. Any minor hurdle in communication will lead to a problematic situation, especially in high-pressure environments.

Hence, impeccable verbal and nonverbal communication techniques are essential in a nursing role. It becomes all the more critical when it comes to listening, tracking, and presenting information related to a patient. Besides verbal and nonverbal skills, nurses must stay updated with the latest technological tools, such as healthcare software. This is necessary to facilitate information transfer to the relevant persons. Additionally, good communication skills are necessary to address barriers between nurses and patients or their families. Proactive communication is also important, as patients are usually anxious about their health. They must be provided with precise and reliable information about their health and treatment. From test results to diagnosis and treatment plans, every aspect of information needs to be conveyed explicitly without vagueness.

How can nurses improve their skills to play a more effective role?

Professional Development: A Key to Nursing Success

With rapid advancements in medical knowledge and technology, professional development has become essential to nursing success. As jobs in the nursing sector continue to grow steadily, ongoing education and skill enhancement have become increasingly important for nurses who want to excel in their careers and deliver the highest quality care.

At the national level, employment opportunities for registered nurses have recorded a significant rise. According to the U.S. Bureau of Labor Statistics, jobs in this sector are projected to grow by approximately nine percent over the next decade. This steady growth reflects the expanding demand for healthcare services driven by an aging population, increased chronic health conditions, and broader access to healthcare.

Back in 2020, nurses held around 3.1 million jobs. Approximately 60 percent were employed in hospital settings, while the remaining 40 percent worked in home healthcare services, nursing facilities, physicians' offices, clinics, schools, the military, and other diverse environments.

Given this promising growth, the critical question becomes: how can nurses continuously improve their skills to remain competitive and effective? Here are a few practical strategies to get started:

1. Commit to Lifelong Learning

Nurses who have earned a Bachelor of Science in Nursing (BSN) or an equivalent degree already possess a solid foundation of knowledge and skills required to provide safe and effective patient care. However, the learning process must never stop. The healthcare landscape evolves rapidly, and staying current is vital.

If pursuing an additional degree is not feasible, nurses should seek other educational opportunities to continue their professional growth. This could include:

- **Earning Certifications:** Specialized certifications such as Certified Nursing Assistant (CNA), Certified Emergency Nurse (CEN), or wound care certifications can broaden expertise and open doors to new career paths.
- **Attending Workshops and Seminars:** These provide

valuable opportunities to acquire updated knowledge, learn new techniques, and network with peers.

- **Volunteering and Cross-Training:** Gaining experience in different healthcare settings or specialties enhances practical skills and adaptability.

2. Enhance Communication Skills Continuously

As previously discussed, effective communication is a cornerstone of quality healthcare. Yet, developing and maintaining strong communication skills requires ongoing effort and practice.

Nurses should actively seek feedback from colleagues, patients, and supervisors to identify areas for improvement. Participating in role-playing exercises, workshops on cultural competence, and courses in patient education can significantly boost these skills.

Mastering communication not only improves patient outcomes but also fosters better teamwork and collaboration within multidisciplinary healthcare teams.

3. Develop Technological Proficiency

In today's healthcare environment, technology plays a central role. Nurses must be comfortable using electronic health records (EHR), telemedicine platforms, and various medical devices.

Regular training on new healthcare technologies and digital tools will help nurses work more efficiently and reduce errors. Embracing technology also enables nurses to provide more timely and personalized care to patients.

4. Cultivate Leadership and Advocacy Skills

Professional development is not just about clinical skills; leadership and advocacy are equally important. Nurses who develop these skills can influence positive change in healthcare policies, improve patient safety standards, and mentor junior staff.

Engaging in leadership courses, joining nursing associations, or taking on committee roles within healthcare institutions can help nurses build confidence and expand their impact beyond direct patient care.

The key to the successful delivery of services is based on the ability to be a good listener. This requires an attentive role and the ability not to be distracted in the heat of the moment. A feeling of distraction or rush makes nursing tasks challenging to manage and sends a negative message to patients and their families.

When trying to boost this primary skill, nurses need to adopt a proactive approach where they learn to be good listeners and can convey information based on the patient's perspective. This is because a nurse's role also encompasses educating and counseling patients from their perspective. In this regard, learning to communicate with patients based on their culture, opinions, and concerns is necessary.

5. Learn to adopt a patient-centric approach

At the heart of healthcare services lies the philosophy of adopting a patient-centric approach and focusing on the people. Since nurses have to multitask and are deeply involved with their responsibilities, it is expected that they may need to catch up on their fundamental responsibility of interacting with their patients.

The quality that a nurse must learn over time is to connect with people. The ability to give undivided attention to patients makes the difference. The main skill that must be learned is always to focus on maintaining and staying attentive to patients and on ways to improve their lives.

18: Life Stories of An R.N. Treating Dialysis Patient

Starting as a registered nurse, I have acquired immense experience in the field of dialysis, especially regarding the various technicalities surrounding the treatment protocol and its practical implementation. My inspiration and desire to serve in this specialized area stem from early family experiences that profoundly shaped my attitude toward kidney disease and its treatment.

As a young lady, I spent much of my early years living with my grandparents. Since my parents worked abroad and I remained behind to complete my education, my grandparents became an integral part of my daily life and upbringing. However, much to my concern, I observed that my grandparents led very sedentary lives, which eventually influenced my understanding of chronic illness and preventive health.

While I had studied in school that many diseases are common in old age, I was troubled by some of the choices they made that worsened their health risks. Despite being affluent and well-off—able to afford any food they desired—the disturbing part was their reluctance to engage in physical exercise. Although they followed relatively healthy dietary habits, neither made any meaningful effort to stay active or lose excess weight. Regular visits to the gym or participation in physical activities were dismissed or avoided

Uncovering the Root Causes of Dialysis Needs

altogether.

Adding to their health challenges, my grandfather was a heavy smoker, consuming about a packet of cigarettes daily. Since my junior years in school, I had already learned about the serious health risks associated with smoking, and witnessing this habit firsthand stirred a deep distrust and concern within me. I understood that such unhealthy behaviors severely affect a person's quality of life and increase vulnerability to chronic diseases, including those affecting kidney function.

These early observations left a lasting impression on me. I realized that knowledge alone was not enough—habits, lifestyle choices, and support systems play a critical role in health outcomes. My grandparents' experiences fueled my determination to pursue nursing with a focus on kidney health and dialysis treatment. I wanted to contribute not only to the clinical care of patients but also to their education and empowerment to adopt healthier lifestyles.

Working with dialysis patients has reinforced this understanding daily. I witness how managing kidney disease requires both medical expertise and compassionate encouragement to help patients embrace necessary lifestyle changes. It is a challenging but deeply rewarding field where technical skills blend with empathy and patient education to improve lives.

My grandpa's reluctance to visit a healthcare facility for regular check-ups aggravated the matter further. After some time, my grandpa started complaining of signs and symptoms that I later learned, as a Registered Nurse, were related to kidney disease. These symptoms included muscle cramps, nausea, frequent vomiting, fatigue, and shortness of breath. He was referred to a dialysis unit for treatment. However, unfortunately, the persistent signs that were now being observed were indicators of a much larger problem that had aggravated over a long time but had gone unobserved earlier. One day, following some time in the dialysis unit, I lost my grandpa.

I had performed hemodialysis treatment before my grandfather succumbed to exsanguination while undergoing dialysis. However, this tragedy shaped my future life. Being a registered nurse, I know how crucial dialysis is for treating kidney patients. Without routine dialysis, patients—particularly the elderly and those with renal failure—can become lethargic, confused, bloated, and experience skin thickness and color changes. They may find moving difficult due to fluid retention near their joints. Patients can and will suffer if a facility cannot meet their demands and fails to provide treatment even for a day or two. Death and excruciating anguish could be the end outcome.

Even though dialysis is a life-saving treatment, the procedure is often accompanied by numerous challenges that complicate the patient's journey. Improving health outcomes through dialysis requires not only advanced medical care but also strength and

Uncovering the Root Causes of Dialysis Needs

resilience from both patients and their families. This dual support system plays a crucial role in navigating the complexities of the treatment process.

Hemodialysis can be performed in different settings—either at an independent dialysis center or within a hospital's dialysis unit. Regardless of the location, the commitment required from patients remains substantial. Typically, patients must attend dialysis sessions about three times per week, with each session lasting between three to four hours. This schedule demands significant time investment and can disrupt patients' daily routines and lifestyles.

Adjusting to the rigorous demands of dialysis is often a difficult and gradual process. Patients face the stark reality of incorporating this intensive treatment into their lives while managing the emotional and physical toll it can impose. The first few weeks or months can be especially challenging, as individuals work to accept their new normal.

Despite the challenges, dialysis remains a critical, life-sustaining therapy that requires consistency and a steadfast approach. Patients must adhere to strict treatment schedules, dietary restrictions, and medication regimens to maximize the therapy's benefits. Support from family members, caregivers, and healthcare professionals is essential to help patients remain motivated and compliant throughout their treatment journey.

Moreover, the psychological impact of dialysis should not be underestimated. Feelings of anxiety, depression, and fatigue are common, making emotional resilience just as important as physical endurance. Nurses and healthcare teams play a vital role in providing holistic care that addresses both the physical and emotional needs of patients.

Due to the challenges I experienced with my family after losing our grandpa, I developed a profound emotional attachment to helping improve patients' lives through the hemodialysis regimen. Frequent hemodialysis is essential for a kidney patient's body to maintain a healthy fluid and mineral balance and control blood pressure.

The sad part is that the dialysis treatment process is often marred by errors that can be avoided with education. I found this career very satisfying, with the role varying widely. Over time, I learned that my role as a renal nurse required being more than just a technical expert with a lot of knowledge and skills. I needed to simultaneously perform the roles of facilitator, mentor, caregiver, educator, and advocate. It is not just about providing dialysis therapy as ordered by the doctor. Rather, the role envisions a broader concept where I am bound to serve as an educator, advising patients on their illness, diet, medications, and other aspects. Most importantly, it is about working as a responsible team member and collaborating with related staff to ensure compliance with treatment.

Uncovering the Root Causes of Dialysis Needs

Starting my career as an RN at Chinatown Dialysis Center in New York, U.S., in 2009, the role of a qualified renal nurse with a nursing license has proven very rewarding. With its enormous demands, adjusting to the new position and setting was challenging and disheartening to see your skills specified in one practice area. However, with time, the role has proven very satisfying. Most importantly, renal nursing being a dynamic field offers plenty of room for growth and improvement, albeit with its share of challenges.

An important aspect I observed throughout my experience working with dialysis patients was the necessity to engage with them over the long term. This long-term involvement presented a unique and complex challenge: I had to carefully maintain professional boundaries while fully embracing my responsibilities. Striking the right balance between professionalism and empathy became crucial, especially as many patients and their families grew to regard our dialysis team as an extended family. Building these meaningful relationships required trust, respect, and consistent communication, all while upholding ethical standards that protect both the patient and the healthcare provider.

Ensuring patient compliance with the treatment protocol emerged as another significant challenge in my role. Patients must adhere strictly to dietary restrictions, fluid intake limits, and medication regimens to optimize the benefits of dialysis. Educating patients and their families about the critical importance of compliance is essential, but it is not always easy. At times, patients may become non-compliant—whether due to misunderstanding, emotional fatigue, or a desire to maintain a semblance of normalcy. Such behavior can severely jeopardize their health, increasing the risk of hospitalization and other life-threatening complications. The possibility that non-compliance might lead to death underscores the gravity and responsibility inherent in the nurse's role as an educator, motivator, and advocate.

Working on such a demanding schedule inevitably exposed me to caregiver fatigue. The physical and emotional toll of caring for chronically ill patients on a daily basis is considerable and cannot be underestimated. It is a burden shared by many in the healthcare profession, and addressing caregiver fatigue requires self-awareness, support, and resilience. Equally important is recognizing that the patients themselves face significant mental health challenges. Dialysis often restricts their lifestyle choices, affecting their independence and emotional well-being. The need of the hour is for nurses to demonstrate patience, compassion, and an informed, holistic approach to improve not just the physical but also the psychological health of dialysis patients.

One of the most rewarding aspects of being a renal nurse is the opportunity to learn about patients beyond their medical conditions. This deepened understanding allows renal nurses to become integral

Uncovering the Root Causes of Dialysis Needs

parts of their patients' lives. From my experience, creating a supportive, welcoming environment where the dialysis team, patients, and families all feel at home fosters a sense of community and belonging that is invaluable in improving treatment outcomes. This familial atmosphere encourages patients to adhere better to their protocols and helps alleviate some of the isolation and anxiety that often accompany chronic illness.

Moreover, helping dialysis patients maintain an active and healthy lifestyle brings an incredible sense of accomplishment. Knowing that my efforts contribute directly to saving lives and enhancing quality of life is profoundly fulfilling. These moments of success, however small, reaffirm the purpose behind the long hours and emotional demands of the job. In short, my career as a renal nurse has been deeply gratifying. It has not only boosted my professional self-esteem and satisfaction but has also enriched my personal growth by allowing me to witness resilience, hope, and the human spirit in its most vulnerable and courageous moments.

19: NxStage Home Hemodialysis

A Brief Overview of the NxStage Machine and In-Center Dialysis

The NxStage machine is a portable home dialysis device designed to perform hemodialysis in the comfort of a patient's own home. It offers a flexible alternative to traditional in-center dialysis by requiring minimal modifications to home electrical and plumbing systems. The machine is user-friendly, making it easier for patients and caregivers to manage treatments with proper training. NxStage also allows for more frequent dialysis sessions, which can lead to better overall health outcomes and reduced strain on the body.

In-center dialysis refers to treatments administered at a specialized dialysis facility under the supervision of trained medical staff. Patients typically visit the center three times per week for several hours per session. In-center dialysis ensures professional monitoring, immediate access to medical intervention in case of complications, and support from healthcare staff who manage all aspects of the treatment process.

Is Home Dialysis Better than In-Center?

Home hemodialysis offers several potential benefits compared to in-center dialysis. Patients have the flexibility to schedule sessions at times that suit their daily routines, including overnight or more frequent shorter treatments. This flexibility often leads to improved quality of life and a greater sense of independence.

Additionally, home dialysis allows patients to experience the comfort and privacy of their own homes, which can reduce stress and anxiety associated with frequent trips to a dialysis center. More frequent or longer dialysis sessions at home can also improve overall health outcomes, including better blood pressure control, reduced fluid buildup, and improved energy levels.

However, home dialysis requires patients or caregivers to be trained to operate the equipment safely and manage treatments effectively. While it offers freedom and convenience, it also demands responsibility and commitment. For some patients, in-center dialysis remains the preferred choice due to the constant supervision, immediate access to medical professionals, and social interaction with staff and fellow patients.

NxStage System One S Home Machine Operation Mechanism

The NxStage System One S is the first portable hemodialysis system specifically cleared by the FDA for home use. Its compact design, approximately one foot tall, offers patients unparalleled freedom and mobility, allowing them to continue their therapy while traveling. The machine is designed for simplicity, with an intuitive interface that makes operation easy to understand and follow, even for patients with minimal technical experience.

When combined with the **NxStage PureFlow SL Dialysis**

Preparation System, the process of creating dialysis fluid is greatly simplified. The system uses ordinary tap water to generate dialysis solution, eliminating the need for specialized water treatment infrastructure required by conventional hemodialysis systems. This innovation allows for a seamless home setup without costly or complex plumbing modifications.

The NxStage System One S is widely adopted by leading hospitals across the United States due to its versatility and patient-centered design. The machine provides a broad range of flow rates, enabling treatments to be customized to individual patient needs. It features a unique **volumetric balancing system** that ensures precise fluid management without the use of scales, reducing the risk of alarms associated with traditional scale-based systems. Additionally, effluent drains directly into an open drain, eliminating interruptions caused by emptying waste bags and reducing staff workload while maintaining treatment accuracy.

Patient safety and ease of use are central to the NxStage design. The operation requires no complex controls, and training for patients and caregivers is straightforward and streamlined. The disposable cartridge system minimizes blood-air interfaces, which helps prevent filter clotting and reduces the risk of complications. Moreover, the machine requires no special electrical or plumbing modifications, making it highly adaptable for a variety of home environments.

Uncovering the Root Causes of Dialysis Needs

Comparison: Home Frequent Hemodialysis vs. Conventional Thrice-Weekly Dialysis

Home frequent hemodialysis provides several notable advantages over conventional thrice-weekly in-center dialysis. Research indicates that performing dialysis **five to seven times per week** significantly improves overall health outcomes, enhances quality of life, and increases survival rates. More frequent treatments help the body maintain a more consistent balance of fluids, electrolytes, and toxins, reducing the strain on the heart and other organs.

One of the key benefits of home dialysis is **patient autonomy**. Once trained, patients can manage their treatments independently without relying on dialysis center staff. This independence allows for greater flexibility in scheduling, enabling patients to fit dialysis sessions around their personal and professional routines. Performing dialysis at home also eliminates the need for frequent travel to a dialysis center, reducing stress, time commitment, and transportation costs.

In contrast, conventional thrice-weekly dialysis often leads to **significant fluid and toxin buildup** between sessions. This accumulation can cause uncomfortable symptoms such as swelling, high blood pressure, fatigue, and shortness of breath. More frequent dialysis at home mitigates these issues, helping patients feel more energetic, stable, and healthier overall.

Home frequent hemodialysis also offers psychological and

emotional benefits. Patients report a greater sense of control over their treatment, reduced anxiety, and improved mental well-being. Being in the familiar environment of their own home adds comfort and privacy, enhancing the overall treatment experience.

Ultimately, the most important factor in dialysis therapy is ensuring the patient receives **adequate dialysis** to maintain optimal health. Proper treatment helps reduce hospital visits, prevent complications, and extend life expectancy. The nephrologist determines the dialysis prescription based on individual factors such as fluid accumulation between sessions, remaining kidney function, body weight, and toxin levels. By tailoring treatment to each patient's needs, home frequent hemodialysis can deliver superior clinical outcomes compared to conventional thrice-weekly dialysis.

Advantages and Risks of Hemodialysis at an In-Center or Skilled Nursing Facility

In-center hemodialysis is performed at a specialized dialysis center under the supervision of trained medical staff. Patients typically attend **three sessions per week**, each lasting **three to four hours**.

Advantages:

- **Professional oversight:** Trained staff monitor patients throughout the procedure, ensuring safety and immediate response to complications.

Uncovering the Root Causes of Dialysis Needs

- **Access to diagnostics:** Laboratory tests and patient assessments are readily available, allowing clinicians to track health status closely.

- **Structured environment:** The predictable routine can help patients manage their treatment schedule.

- **Social and recreational opportunities:** Patients can relax, read, or interact with others during sessions, which can provide emotional support.

Risks and Drawbacks:

- **Fixed schedules:** Patients must adhere to the center's timetable, limiting flexibility and personal control.

- **Travel requirements:** Frequent trips to the center can be inconvenient and exhausting, particularly for elderly or mobility-limited patients.

- **Dietary restrictions:** Less frequent dialysis necessitates strict adherence to fluid and dietary limits.

- **Limited privacy:** Shared spaces may restrict personal comfort and confidentiality.

Advantages and Risks of Hemodialysis at Home

Home hemodialysis offers **greater flexibility and independence**, allowing patients to schedule treatments according to their personal routines. This flexibility often leads to reduced stress and improved mental well-being. By eliminating travel to a dialysis center, patients save significant time, **on average up to 52 days per year** when accounting for travel, waiting, and recovery.

Additional Benefits:

- **Faster recovery:** Home dialysis patients typically experience shorter recovery times compared to the eight-hour recovery period often required after in-center sessions.

- **Reduced medication reliance:** Frequent home dialysis can improve fluid and toxin control, potentially reducing the need for medications such as blood pressure or phosphate-lowering drugs.

- **Improved transplant eligibility:** Better overall health and stability can enhance a patient's suitability for kidney transplantation.

- **Travel convenience:** Portable machines like the **NxStage System One** allow patients to continue therapy while traveling, reducing the need to arrange alternative dialysis options.

Risks and Considerations:

- **Reduced supervision:** Treatments are performed without direct medical oversight, requiring patients and caregivers to be vigilant and well-trained.

- **Increased vascular access use:** Frequent dialysis can increase the risk of infections, clotting, or access-related complications.

- **Responsibility and commitment:** Patients must follow strict protocols for machine operation, hygiene, and monitoring for potential issues.

Overall, both in-center and home dialysis have distinct advantages and risks. The choice depends on the patient's medical condition, lifestyle, support system, and personal preferences. Collaboration with a nephrologist is essential to determine the safest and most effective treatment approach.

Reasons to Choose NxStage: Is It the Future of Home Hemodialysis?

There are many reasons to choose NxStage. It offers numerous advantages for those who want to make home hemodialysis a reality.

Most importantly, NxStage is a portable hemodialysis system. It comes with an interface that is simple to install and use at home. This machine offers great flexibility, making it possible to realize the dream of home hemodialysis. It has been specifically designed for patients, providing an easy-to-use interface tailored to their needs.

The main advantage of NxStage is that it allows frequent and flexible therapy at home. Patients can schedule treatments according to their preferences, giving them more control and independence in managing their health.

As noted earlier, the machine requires little to no home modifications. It can be used in any part of the home without difficulty.

NxStage is also designed for portability. It can be moved easily and provides flexibility when traveling, with two options for dialysate supply: bags or the PureFlow SL system.

Another key feature is its ease of handling. The treatment process uses a drop-in cartridge, which simplifies setup and cleanup. After each treatment, the cartridge can be removed and the device quickly wiped down. Each cartridge includes an integrated dialyzer and bloodlines, ensuring an easy and reliable setup. The design minimizes the risk of user errors that can occur with dialyzer connections and reduces the chance of contamination at touch-points.

NxStage represents the future of dialysis. It is the first portable hemodialysis system cleared in the United States for home use. It supports both solo hemodialysis (performed during waking hours) and nocturnal hemodialysis (when the patient and caregiver can sleep).

By revolutionizing dialysis treatment, NxStage allows patients to safely undergo therapy at home. Its compact size and portability also provide patients with greater freedom to travel, making treatment more adaptable to modern lifestyles.

20: The Future Of Your Health Is In Your Hands And Evolving Modern Dialysis Technology Is Around The Corner

Improvement in Dialysis Treatment Outcomes

In recent years, dialysis treatment has experienced remarkable advancements, leading to significantly better patient outcomes. For much of the previous century, mortality rates among dialysis patients remained largely unchanged, despite the growing number of individuals requiring treatment. However, in the past few decades, mortality rates for maintenance dialysis patients have declined sharply, representing a major milestone in nephrology and renal care. This improvement is considered a significant achievement, though it also highlights the ongoing need to build upon these advances to further enhance survival and quality of life.

A key driver of this progress has been the substantial investment in healthcare research and innovation. Rising healthcare costs have coincided with increased funding for studies focused on improving treatment efficacy, patient safety, and long-term outcomes. Research efforts have documented numerous technological and procedural innovations, which have directly contributed to better dialysis care.

The development and adoption of new medical technologies,

particularly in the early part of the last century, have played a pivotal role in transforming dialysis therapy. These innovations include more efficient dialysis machines, improved vascular access techniques, and enhanced monitoring systems, all of which have collectively boosted treatment quality.

Early attempts at managed care, although initially limited in effectiveness, provided a foundation for evidence-based practices in dialysis. By focusing on systematic improvements in care delivery, such as standardized treatment protocols, patient monitoring, and integrated care pathways, the field has been able to reduce complications, optimize dialysis schedules, and improve patient outcomes.

The Gloom Surrounding Dialysis Treatment is Over

End-stage renal disease (ESRD) is a major public health challenge, affecting approximately 700,000 Americans, of whom around 400,000 rely on life-saving hemodialysis. While hemodialysis is essential for sustaining life, it can impose a significant physical, emotional, and psychological burden on patients. Many individuals experience fatigue, discomfort, and limitations in daily activities, contributing to a reduced quality of life.

Studies consistently show that, when compared to patients with other chronic illnesses, such as cancer, congestive heart failure, or chronic obstructive pulmonary disease, hemodialysis patients report the lowest scores in health-related quality of life (HrQOL). These low scores are associated with challenges in performing self-care, adhering to treatment regimens, and maintaining overall well-being. Poor HrQOL can also contribute to worse clinical outcomes, including higher hospitalization rates and increased morbidity.

However, recent innovations in dialysis treatment, including home hemodialysis, portable machines like the NxStage System One, and more frequent treatment schedules, are helping to transform this bleak outlook. Patients now have greater flexibility, independence, and control over their therapy, allowing them to better manage their health and improve overall quality of life. By reducing travel, fatigue, and treatment-related stress, these advancements are helping to lift the historical gloom surrounding dialysis treatment and offer patients a more hopeful and empowered path forward.

What the Pandemic Meant for Dialysis Treatment

The COVID-19 pandemic brought sweeping changes in healthcare practices. From mask-wearing and hand hygiene to the widespread adoption of telehealth, patients and providers adapted quickly. For dialysis, the pandemic accelerated the shift toward home-based care, redefining how treatment is delivered.

The home healthcare market, valued at $229 billion in 2020, is projected to grow by nearly 8% annually. This growth has revolutionized the healthcare landscape. While critics note that patients may lose certain in-person perks, the benefits far outweigh the drawbacks. Home-based healthcare offers flexibility, control, and autonomy.

Dialysis, once considered too complex for home treatment, has also embraced this transformation. Patients now see the benefits of avoiding rigid clinic schedules, lengthy travel, and exposure to infectious environments. Home dialysis empowers patients to live more fully, aligning their treatment with their personal routines and lifestyle choices.

Dialysis Treatment: Hope with Room for Improvement

Despite lingering skepticism about dialysis, much of it arises from the recognition that improvements are still needed, rather than from evidence of failure. Compared to the 1960s, kidney patients today are living longer, healthier, and more fulfilling lives. They also enjoy better access to healthcare and a wider range of treatment options.

Still, challenges remain. The need for further progress is undeniable, but it should not overshadow the significant accomplishments achieved in recent decades.

For the 37 million Americans living with kidney disease, and for their families, dialysis represents new hope. While kidney disease remains a silent killer that exacts a heavy toll on patients, families, and the healthcare system, early and effective treatment can slow its progression. Without intervention, kidney disease may advance to end stage renal disease, requiring dialysis or a transplant. However, with continued innovation and timely treatment, patients can look forward to longer, healthier lives.

Though in the past, the first year of undergoing dialysis treatment was challenging for patients due to the complex needs associated with this treatment, the situation has improved. The number of patients suffering from kidney failure has declined, and those undergoing dialysis are now able to live longer lives. In addition, less time needs to be spent in hospitals. Overall, these advances have saved lives and billions of dollars, allowing the healthcare system to invest in other directions.

Increased home dialysis will be the new norm in the future

Home dialysis is being dubbed the new norm, and rightly so, because it offers a convenient and effective solution to an ever-growing problem. Half a million Americans are already being treated with dialysis three times a week for four hours per session, a schedule that places immense physical, emotional, and logistical burdens on patients and their families. Shifting the focus to home dialysis could dramatically improve quality of life while simultaneously reducing strain on hospitals and outpatient centers. Current in-clinic methods not only increase the healthcare system's cost but also add to patients' difficulties, including frequent transportation, missed work or school, and prolonged exposure to potentially stressful clinical environments.

Experts are constantly aiming to find safer and more efficient ways to improve dialysis treatment. Innovations such as portable dialysis machines, telehealth monitoring, and patient-friendly training programs are paving the way for a more accessible home-based model. However, barriers remain, including the need to ensure that dialysis providers are relieved of staffing and supply responsibilities, the costs of equipment and home setup, and the need for ongoing patient support. These challenges must be addressed in a comprehensive system designed to serve kidney patients effectively while lowering the burden on the healthcare system.

The COVID-19 pandemic has further accelerated the shift toward home dialysis. Kidney patients are particularly vulnerable due to weakened immune systems, making exposure to hospital or clinic environments especially dangerous. Even when precautions are strictly followed, a hospital setting inherently carries higher risk. Staffing shortages during the pandemic forced clinics to treat patients with fewer personnel and limited space, magnifying the risk of infection. Home dialysis eliminates many of these exposure risks, providing a safer and more controlled environment for treatment.

Despite these advantages, adoption remains strikingly low. Statistics indicate that almost 30% of dialysis patients are clinically eligible for home dialysis, yet only 2% currently receive treatment at home. This gap highlights a significant opportunity to improve patient outcomes, enhance independence, and reduce systemic costs. Expanding access to home dialysis, through education, training, financial support, and infrastructure investment, is therefore a critical step toward modernizing kidney care and empowering patients to take control of their treatment.

Moreover, studies have shown that home dialysis can lead to better clinical outcomes, including improved blood pressure control, fewer hospitalizations, and enhanced survival rates. Patients often report higher satisfaction and an improved sense of autonomy, as they can schedule sessions around daily life and maintain a more normal routine. With growing technological advancements, including smart dialysis machines that monitor treatment in real time and provide remote clinical support, home dialysis is becoming not only feasible but preferable for many patients.

The future of kidney care lies in empowering patients, reducing systemic burdens, and leveraging technology to bring effective treatment into the home. The transition to home dialysis is not just a trend, it is an essential evolution in healthcare, offering safety, convenience, and a higher quality of life for millions of Americans.

Uncovering the Root Causes of Dialysis Needs

What the future holds for dialysis treatment

Technological advancements and innovations are poised to redefine the future of dialysis treatment. Current dialysis methods, while life-saving, are expected to evolve, or even become obsolete, replaced by approaches that offer more effective and personalized care with improved health outcomes. Smaller, mobile-based technologies are anticipated to provide metabolic support, potentially allowing patients to maintain a more normal lifestyle. Looking further ahead, wearable devices or even fully automated artificial kidneys could take over the body's metabolic functions, performing the work of natural kidneys in real time.

While these developments may sound like science fiction, they are rapidly becoming achievable through advances in biomedical engineering, materials science, and digital health. Mobile sensors capable of monitoring parameters such as food intake, hydration, and lifestyle habits are already in development, promising to revolutionize how kidney function is managed and how treatment plans are personalized. Furthermore, experts foresee the integrated use of 3D-printed tissue and intelligent biomaterials to replicate kidney design and function, potentially offering solutions that mimic natural organ performance with unprecedented precision.

Ongoing research and early successes in these fields make such possibilities increasingly realistic. Although the exact form of kidney treatment in the next decade remains uncertain, the trajectory points toward a future where dialysis patients can lead healthier, more autonomous lives. These innovations hold the promise of significantly improved survival rates, reduced dependence on in-clinic care, and a higher quality of life, transforming kidney treatment from a burdensome necessity into a seamless, integrated part of daily living.

PART II:
Transforming Healthcare

Introduction

Dialysis care is complex and requires a coordinated approach to address the diverse medical, social, and emotional needs of patients. Managing these patients is not solely the responsibility of nephrologists or nurses; it involves a wide range of healthcare professionals, each contributing specialized expertise. This underscores the significance of interdisciplinary collaboration, where professionals such as dietitians, social workers, pharmacists, and psychologists work alongside physicians and nurses to provide holistic care. However, collaboration alone is not enough. Effective communication and coordination are essential to ensure patients do not experience fragmented care. Here, case managers play a central role. By serving as liaisons among healthcare team members, they ensure that information is shared accurately and timely, treatment goals are aligned, and patients receive consistent care. The impact of this model extends beyond better communication; it has the potential to reduce hospitalization rates, improve health outcomes, and enhance the overall well-being of dialysis patients.

Importance of Case Management

Case management is a vital component of modern healthcare delivery, especially for patients with chronic conditions such as kidney disease. Case managers serve as advocates, helping patients navigate the often confusing healthcare system. Many dialysis patients face challenges such as limited mobility, financial stress, transportation barriers, and comorbid illnesses. Without guidance, these obstacles can prevent them from accessing the care they need. Case managers step in to bridge these gaps.

By coordinating care across different specialties and care settings—dialysis centers, hospitals, primary care clinics, and community resources—they promote continuity of care. This reduces duplication of services, prevents gaps in treatment, and ensures patients follow through with their care plans. Additionally, case managers engage in proactive assessment and intervention. They identify potential risks to health outcomes, such as medication non-adherence, dietary challenges, or social determinants of health like housing insecurity or lack of family support. Addressing these issues early can significantly improve the patient's ability to manage their condition.

Role of Case Managers

The role of case managers extends beyond logistics. They conduct comprehensive assessments that evaluate patients' medical, social, and psychological needs. Based on these assessments, they design individualized care plans tailored to each patient's circumstances. For example, a patient struggling with transportation may have appointments scheduled around accessible services, while another may require counseling support to cope with the stress of long-term dialysis.

Case managers also play a crucial role in coordinating appointments and facilitating communication between healthcare professionals. They monitor progress, track lab results, and adjust care plans as needed. Equally important, they serve as educators, providing patients with knowledge about their condition, treatment options, and self-management techniques. By empowering patients to understand and take responsibility for their health, case managers foster confidence, independence, and resilience.

Benefits of Case Management

The benefits of case management in dialysis care are far-reaching. One of the most significant is the reduction of hospitalization rates. Many hospital admissions among dialysis patients are preventable with proper monitoring, early intervention, and preventive care. Case managers identify health concerns before they escalate into emergencies, thereby reducing costly hospital stays.

Medication management is another critical benefit. Dialysis patients often take multiple medications, which can lead to confusion, missed doses, or harmful drug interactions. Case managers work closely with patients to simplify regimens, encourage adherence, and monitor side effects, ensuring optimal therapeutic outcomes.

Finally, case management greatly improves patient satisfaction.

Patients who feel supported and understood are more likely to engage with their healthcare providers and comply with treatment recommendations. Personalized guidance and advocacy enhance their overall healthcare experience and promote a stronger sense of empowerment and well-being.

Comprehensive Care Planning in Dialysis

Tailoring Care to Individual Needs

Comprehensive care planning is a cornerstone of effective dialysis management, ensuring that every patient's unique needs are identified and addressed. Dialysis patients often face not only the physical burden of kidney failure but also psychological, social, and financial challenges. Case managers play a critical role in developing individualized care plans that respond to these multifaceted needs.

A **holistic assessment** is the first step in this process. Case managers evaluate patients' physical conditions, comorbidities, mental health, living environments, and social support systems. This broad assessment allows for the identification of potential barriers to care, such as difficulties in medication adherence, transportation challenges, or emotional distress linked to chronic illness.

Once these challenges are identified, case managers design **personalized interventions** aimed at improving the patient's overall quality of life. These interventions may include strategies for symptom management, mental health counseling, lifestyle modifications, and educational programs to enhance self-management skills. For example, a patient struggling with dietary restrictions may benefit from nutrition counseling with a dietitian, while another facing depression might be referred to psychological support services.

Central to this process is **multidisciplinary collaboration**. Comprehensive care plans are not created in isolation but developed in partnership with the broader dialysis care team, including nephrologists, nurses, dietitians, and social workers. Each professional contributes expertise, ensuring that care delivery is coordinated, efficient, and aligned with the patient's goals. By working together, the team can provide a seamless and comprehensive approach that addresses the whole person rather than focusing solely on their disease.

Ensuring Continuity of Care

Equally important to the success of dialysis care is the ability to maintain continuity across different settings and stages of treatment. Case managers act as key coordinators to ensure that patients do not experience gaps or disruptions in their care journey.

One vital responsibility is **transition management**. Dialysis patients frequently move between care settings—for example, from

Uncovering the Root Causes of Dialysis Needs

hospital back to home, or from in-center dialysis to home-based dialysis modalities. These transitions can be overwhelming for patients and their families if not carefully managed. Case managers step in to coordinate follow-up appointments, arrange transportation, and prepare patients with the resources and knowledge they need to adapt to new care environments. By doing so, they reduce the risk of complications and readmissions.

Case managers also excel in **communication facilitation**. They serve as liaisons between patients and the healthcare team, ensuring that critical information is accurately communicated and that care plans are effectively implemented. This role is particularly vital in dialysis, where treatment regimens are complex and require continuous monitoring and adjustment. Clear and timely communication fosters trust and prevents misunderstandings that could compromise care.

Finally, case managers provide **resource navigation** to connect patients with community-based programs, financial assistance, and social support services. Dialysis treatment often comes with significant out-of-pocket costs, lifestyle disruptions, and emotional strain. By linking patients to support groups, counseling services, or financial aid programs, case managers help alleviate burdens and promote overall well-being.

Empowering Patients for Self-Management

One of the most powerful tools in transforming healthcare is patient education, and in dialysis care, case managers play a central role in this process. Patients with kidney disease often find themselves overwhelmed by the complexity of their condition, the intensity of treatment regimens, and the lifestyle adjustments required. Case managers step in to provide clear, accessible, and tailored **disease education**. They explain the causes and progression of kidney disease, the purpose and process of dialysis, and the available treatment options, whether in-center hemodialysis, home hemodialysis, or peritoneal dialysis.

Beyond treatment explanations, case managers emphasize **self-care strategies** that empower patients to participate actively in their care. Patients learn how to track their fluid intake, monitor blood pressure, and recognize early warning signs of complications such as infection or fluid overload. This knowledge not only reduces fear and confusion but also builds confidence, enabling patients to feel more in control of their condition.

Lifestyle Modification: Promoting Healthier Living

Managing kidney disease effectively requires significant lifestyle adjustments, and case managers serve as guides in this critical area. They help patients adopt **renal-friendly diets** that limit sodium, potassium, and phosphorus while ensuring adequate protein intake.

Uncovering the Root Causes of Dialysis Needs

Nutrition counseling, often delivered in collaboration with dietitians, helps patients make realistic food choices that fit their preferences and cultural backgrounds.

In addition to dietary changes, case managers encourage **regular physical activity**, tailored to each patient's capabilities and health status. Even moderate activities such as walking or stretching can improve cardiovascular health, reduce fatigue, and boost emotional well-being. Stress management is another vital area, as dialysis patients often experience anxiety or depression. Case managers may introduce coping strategies such as mindfulness, breathing exercises, or referrals to mental health services. By addressing these lifestyle factors, case managers help optimize both health outcomes and quality of life.

Self-Management Support: Encouraging Independence

Self-management is the cornerstone of long-term success in dialysis care. Case managers teach patients **practical skills** for managing their treatment at home, such as recording dialysis logs, caring for vascular access sites, and maintaining hygiene to prevent infection. Patients are also coached to monitor symptoms like swelling, fatigue, or changes in appetite, enabling them to respond quickly to potential complications.

This proactive approach reduces dependence on emergency care and hospitalizations while fostering a sense of independence. Patients who can confidently manage their care are more likely to adhere to treatment and feel empowered in their health journey.

Improving Treatment Adherence

Medication Management: Ensuring Safe and Effective Use

Dialysis patients often take multiple medications, including phosphate binders, antihypertensives, and supplements. Case managers provide **medication education**, explaining the purpose, correct dosage, timing, and possible side effects of each drug. They also collaborate with patients to overcome barriers such as cost, side effects, or forgetfulness. Strategies may include simplifying regimens, setting reminders, or coordinating with pharmacists for easier access to prescriptions.

Treatment Compliance: Encouraging Consistency in Dialysis

Consistent attendance at dialysis sessions is critical for survival, yet patients may struggle with fatigue, transportation issues, or lack of motivation. Case managers monitor attendance, provide reminders, and address obstacles directly. They also offer **emotional encouragement**, reminding patients of the importance of adherence in preventing complications and maintaining quality of life.

Supporting Lifestyle Modifications: Sustaining Long-Term Health

Finally, case managers reinforce **healthy lifestyle habits** that directly impact dialysis effectiveness. Encouraging patients to follow dietary restrictions, stay active, and avoid harmful behaviors such as smoking or alcohol use strengthens overall treatment outcomes. These modifications, though challenging, are made more achievable with ongoing guidance, encouragement, and accountability from case managers.

Amplifying Patient Voices

Case managers serve as advocates for patients by ensuring they understand and exercise their rights as healthcare consumers. Many dialysis patients are unaware of their entitlements, which may result in missed opportunities for involvement in their care. Case managers provide education on **patients' rights**, including the right to participate actively in treatment decisions, access medical records, and receive respectful, nondiscriminatory care. This education empowers patients to become active partners rather than passive recipients of treatment.

In addition, case managers play an essential role in **navigating the healthcare system**. Dialysis care often requires interaction with multiple providers, insurance companies, and support services, all of which can be confusing and stressful. Case managers simplify this process by helping patients understand insurance coverage, resolve billing issues, and access specialty care such as cardiology, ophthalmology, or mental health services. By offering this support, case managers reduce frustration and ensure that patients obtain the resources necessary for effective care.

Perhaps most importantly, case managers focus on **empowering patients** to make informed decisions. They provide reliable information, guidance, and encouragement so patients feel confident asserting their preferences, asking questions, and voicing concerns. This empowerment strengthens patient autonomy and fosters a sense of control over the dialysis journey.

Driving Excellence in Dialysis Care

Case managers are not only advocates for individual patients but also catalysts for broader healthcare improvements. Their work in **performance monitoring** is vital to ensuring that dialysis programs meet high standards of safety and effectiveness. They track key performance indicators such as infection rates, hospital readmissions, adherence to clinical protocols, and patient satisfaction. This data-driven approach helps identify gaps in care delivery and highlights areas for improvement.

Beyond monitoring, case managers are instrumental in **process optimization**. They collaborate with the interdisciplinary dialysis team to design and implement strategies that streamline workflows, reduce inefficiencies, and minimize errors. For example, they may introduce standardized checklists for infection control, coordinate medication reconciliation processes, or adjust scheduling systems to reduce patient wait times. These initiatives not only enhance the efficiency of care delivery but also improve the overall patient experience.

Patient feedback is another crucial component of quality improvement. Case managers actively solicit input from patients and families about their care experiences, concerns, and preferences. By incorporating this feedback into quality improvement initiatives, case managers ensure that changes in care delivery are patient-centered and responsive to real-world needs. This continuous cycle of monitoring, optimizing, and integrating feedback drives excellence and fosters trust between patients and providers.

Fostering Collaboration for Holistic Care: The Interdisciplinary Dialysis Team Approach

High-quality dialysis care requires the expertise of multiple professionals working together. The **interdisciplinary dialysis team** typically includes nephrologists, nurses, dietitians, social workers, pharmacists, and other specialists. Each team member contributes unique knowledge and skills, from managing clinical protocols to addressing psychosocial challenges.

Case managers are at the heart of this team, facilitating **communication and coordination** among members. They ensure that everyone is aligned in their responsibilities and that patient care is delivered cohesively rather than in fragmented silos. Effective communication prevents duplication of services, reduces errors, and ensures that patients receive consistent information across all providers.

Shared decision-making is another defining feature of the interdisciplinary approach. Case managers encourage **collaboration between patients, families, and providers** in developing care plans that reflect individual goals, preferences, and values. This approach not only enhances patient satisfaction but also results in more realistic, achievable, and sustainable care outcomes.

Comprehensive Assessment

At the heart of personalized care is the initial assessment process. Case managers take time to gather a complete picture of a patient's medical history, current health status, psychosocial needs, and environmental conditions. For instance, understanding whether a patient has supportive family members, reliable transportation to dialysis centers, or access to nutritious food directly informs the type of support they will need. This holistic evaluation goes beyond lab results and medical charts—it identifies the barriers and enablers that affect daily living.

Multidisciplinary Collaboration

Once a patient's profile is established, case managers collaborate with the broader interdisciplinary dialysis team. This includes nephrologists, nurses, dietitians, social workers, and sometimes

Uncovering the Root Causes of Dialysis Needs

mental health professionals. Family members and caregivers are also invited into the conversation to ensure alignment with the patient's values and lifestyle. Through this collaboration, the care plan reflects a collective understanding of medical requirements, psychosocial support, and patient preferences.

Goal Setting with Patients

Care plans are not abstract guidelines; they are goal-oriented roadmaps. Case managers work with patients to establish specific, measurable, achievable, relevant, and time-bound (SMART) goals. For example, a patient may set a goal to lower their blood pressure within three months, improve adherence to fluid restrictions, or increase physical activity to boost energy. These goals provide both direction and motivation, ensuring that care is purposeful and progress can be tracked.

Ongoing Evaluation and Adjustment

Healthcare is dynamic, and so are patients' lives. Case managers conduct regular evaluations to monitor whether patients are meeting their goals. If challenges arise—such as medication side effects, depression, or financial stressors—case managers adjust the plan accordingly. This flexibility ensures that care remains responsive and effective, helping patients stay on track toward improved health outcomes.

Ensuring Safe and Effective Medication Use

Medication management is often one of the most complex aspects of dialysis care. Patients may be prescribed multiple medications for blood pressure, anemia, bone health, and other conditions related to kidney failure. Without careful oversight, the risk of drug-drug interactions, side effects, or poor adherence can compromise treatment outcomes.

Medication Reconciliation

Case managers begin by reviewing patients' complete medication lists. They carefully reconcile discrepancies between what is prescribed, what is dispensed by pharmacies, and what patients are actually taking. This step is essential to prevent errors such as duplicate prescriptions, incorrect dosages, or harmful combinations of drugs.

Supporting Adherence

Even the best medication plan is ineffective if patients struggle with adherence. Case managers provide education about each prescribed drug—how to take it, why it is important, and what potential side effects to watch for. They also emphasize the importance of consistency, explaining how missing doses or altering schedules can jeopardize health. By addressing fears or misconceptions, case managers build trust and encourage adherence.

Collaboration with Providers

Medication management is a team effort. Case managers communicate regularly with nephrologists, pharmacists, and other specialists to coordinate strategies. If a patient experiences side effects or financial difficulties affording prescriptions, the case manager facilitates solutions, such as adjusting dosages, switching medications, or exploring patient assistance programs.

Monitoring and Follow-Up

The role of a case manager does not stop at education and coordination. They also monitor adherence and track treatment outcomes. Follow-up calls, clinic visits, and digital tools may be used to ensure patients are managing their medications correctly. If lapses are identified, supportive interventions are introduced promptly. Through this consistent oversight, case managers help prevent complications and improve the effectiveness of dialysis treatment.

Empowering Patients Through Education

A major goal of case management is to empower patients with knowledge and skills so they can actively participate in their care. This shift from passive recipients of treatment to informed partners in healthcare is transformative, especially for chronic conditions like kidney disease.

Disease Education

Understanding the nature of kidney disease and the role of dialysis is fundamental. Case managers explain, in clear and accessible language, how dialysis works, what symptoms to expect, and how different treatment options affect health. Patients who grasp the "why" behind their treatment are more likely to engage fully and make informed decisions about their care.

Supporting Lifestyle Modifications

Dialysis patients often need to adopt significant lifestyle changes. Case managers provide guidance on following a renal-friendly diet that controls sodium, potassium, and phosphorus intake. They encourage regular physical activity tailored to each patient's capabilities and discuss strategies to manage stress, sleep, and emotional well-being. For example, patients may be advised on how to prepare low-sodium meals or incorporate light exercise into their daily routines. By addressing lifestyle modifications, case managers help patients protect their remaining kidney function and enhance quality of life.

Promoting Treatment Adherence

Beyond medications, dialysis treatment itself requires strict adherence. Patients may miss sessions due to transportation challenges, financial issues, or emotional fatigue. Case managers work closely with patients to identify barriers and develop solutions—arranging reliable transportation, connecting them with social services, or offering emotional support. By tackling these practical challenges, case managers ensure patients remain engaged in their treatment schedules.

Teaching Self-Care Skills

Empowerment also comes from practical skills that patients can apply daily. Case managers teach patients how to monitor fluid intake, measure blood pressure at home, and recognize early signs of complications such as infection or shortness of breath. These skills not only reduce dependence on healthcare providers but also allow patients to act swiftly in emergencies. With these tools, patients gain confidence and become proactive stewards of their own health.

Team Coordination

At the core of this responsibility is the case manager's role as a liaison. They act as a bridge between patients, caregivers, dialysis staff, and external healthcare providers, ensuring that everyone involved in the patient's care is aligned. By sharing vital information—such as medication updates, lab results, or changes in treatment plans—case managers minimize the risk of miscommunication and duplication of effort. This coordination is particularly important in dialysis, where missed details can have significant consequences for patient safety.

Dialysis Champions

Care Coordination Meetings

A key strategy that case managers employ is organizing and facilitating interdisciplinary care meetings. These gatherings bring together members of the healthcare team to review patients' progress, address complications, and adjust treatment strategies as needed. Such meetings foster collaboration, promote consensus-building, and empower every team member to contribute their expertise. Patients and family members are often included, ensuring that care plans reflect shared decision-making and align with personal goals.

Resource Coordination

The challenges faced by dialysis patients often extend beyond clinical needs. Many struggle with financial stress, transportation difficulties, or lack of social support. Case managers help bridge these gaps by connecting patients with community resources, support services, and educational programs. Whether it is linking a patient to financial assistance, arranging reliable transport to dialysis sessions, or enrolling them in educational workshops, resource coordination strengthens both health outcomes and quality of life.

Continuity of Care

For patients transitioning between hospitals, dialysis centers, and home care settings, continuity is essential. Case managers oversee these transitions to ensure care is uninterrupted, safe, and effective.

They coordinate discharge planning, share care summaries across settings, and follow up with patients during transitions. This seamless continuity reduces hospital readmissions, improves safety, and gives patients and families greater confidence in their care journey.

Driving Quality Improvement in Dialysis Care

Case managers are not only patient advocates but also agents of change within dialysis care systems. By focusing on quality improvement, they help raise standards, prevent complications, and promote consistent excellence in care delivery.

Performance Monitoring

Case managers track key performance indicators (KPIs) that reflect the quality and safety of dialysis care. These include dialysis adequacy, vascular access management, infection control, hospitalization rates, and patient satisfaction. By consistently monitoring such indicators, case managers identify trends and highlight areas that require targeted improvement efforts.

Root Cause Analysis

When adverse events or patient safety incidents occur, case managers conduct root cause analyses to uncover underlying issues. For example, if a patient develops a bloodstream infection, the case manager investigates whether it was linked to improper vascular access care, lapses in hygiene, or systemic process failures. This data-driven approach allows for corrective actions that not only resolve the immediate problem but also prevent recurrence in the future.

Best Practice Implementation

Case managers play a key role in integrating evidence-based practices and clinical guidelines into daily care. They work closely with clinical teams to standardize care protocols, streamline workflows, and reinforce practices that are proven to improve patient outcomes. Whether it is implementing updated infection-control measures or promoting new nutritional guidelines, case managers ensure best practices become routine practice.

Patient Feedback and Engagement

Quality improvement must be patient-centered to be meaningful. Case managers actively solicit feedback from patients regarding their experiences, challenges, and expectations. This feedback is then incorporated into quality initiatives, making patients partners in shaping the care they receive. Such engagement not only enhances satisfaction but also fosters trust, reinforcing the idea that healthcare systems value and respect patients' voices.

Psychosocial Support and Counseling

Living with chronic kidney disease and undergoing dialysis can be emotionally overwhelming. Patients often face grief, anxiety, depression, or a profound sense of life disruption. Addressing these psychosocial challenges is just as important as managing physical health, and case managers provide vital support in this dimension.

Emotional Support

Case managers are trained to offer empathetic listening, validation, and encouragement. They provide a safe space for patients to express fears, frustrations, and hopes. This compassionate presence helps patients cope with emotional distress, fosters resilience, and reassures them that they are not navigating their illness alone.

Social Support

Beyond individual counseling, case managers encourage patients to build and maintain social connections. They facilitate engagement with family members, peer mentors, support groups, and community networks. These connections reduce feelings of isolation, promote companionship, and create a sense of belonging. A patient who shares experiences with peers often finds strength and reassurance in knowing others face similar challenges.

Coping Strategies

Case managers also teach patients practical coping mechanisms to manage stress and mood fluctuations. Relaxation techniques such as deep breathing exercises, mindfulness meditation, and guided imagery can help patients remain calm during difficult periods. Additionally, stress management strategies empower patients to balance their emotional well-being alongside the physical demands of dialysis treatment.

Referrals to Mental Health Professionals

While case managers provide frontline support, they also recognize when patients require specialized intervention. They collaborate with psychologists, counselors, social workers, and psychiatrists to arrange comprehensive mental health assessments and therapies. By facilitating timely referrals, case managers ensure patients with complex psychosocial needs receive professional care tailored to their circumstances.

Advocating for Patient Rights

Advocacy is one of the defining responsibilities of case managers. For patients with kidney disease—who often face vulnerability, long-term treatment, and overwhelming choices—having a trusted advocate ensures that their voices are heard and respected in every stage of care.

Patient Advocacy

Case managers stand at the intersection of patient needs and healthcare delivery. They represent patients' interests, preferences, and concerns to healthcare providers, administrators, policymakers, and insurers. This advocacy empowers patients to make informed decisions and ensures their rights are prioritized in a system that can often feel impersonal or intimidating. Whether negotiating for timely appointments, pushing for fair insurance coverage, or ensuring cultural sensitivity in care delivery, case managers give patients the confidence to assert their preferences.

Care Coordination

Advocacy extends beyond individual encounters to broader systems of care. Case managers push for seamless care transitions, equitable treatment, and timely access to services. For example, a dialysis patient discharged from the hospital must quickly reconnect with their dialysis schedule, have updated medication orders, and understand their post-discharge care plan. Case managers coordinate all these moving parts, reducing the likelihood of missed treatments or medication errors. Their efforts improve patient safety, satisfaction, and continuity of care across inpatient, outpatient, and community settings.

Promoting Health Literacy

Patients can only exercise their rights if they understand them. Case managers provide education about healthcare rights, responsibilities, and available options. They help patients decipher medical jargon, explain treatment alternatives, and outline the implications of different decisions. For instance, a patient considering home dialysis may be unaware of the training, equipment, or lifestyle adjustments required. By simplifying this information, case managers equip patients to make choices that align with their values and life circumstances.

Navigating Ethical Dilemmas

Healthcare often presents ethical challenges. Case managers help navigate these dilemmas, ensuring that principles such as autonomy, privacy, confidentiality, and informed consent remain at the forefront. Consider a scenario where a patient refuses a recommended treatment, but family members urge otherwise. The case manager's role is to mediate this conflict, honor the patient's right to autonomy, and ensure decisions are made with respect and dignity. By addressing ethical dilemmas thoughtfully, case managers safeguard the moral integrity of healthcare delivery.

Fostering Collaboration: The Interdisciplinary Approach to Dialysis Care

Dialysis treatment is not a single discipline's responsibility—it requires collaboration across a broad spectrum of healthcare professionals. Case managers ensure that this collaboration is structured, consistent, and effective, preventing the fragmentation of care that can occur in complex medical systems.

Uncovering the Root Causes of Dialysis Needs

Team-Based Care

Case managers work hand in hand with nephrologists, dialysis nurses, dietitians, pharmacists, and social workers to develop holistic care plans. Each professional brings unique expertise: nephrologists manage the medical aspects, dietitians provide nutritional guidance, pharmacists optimize medication safety, and social workers address psychosocial challenges. Case managers weave these contributions together, ensuring that no aspect of patient care is overlooked. This team-based approach provides patients with well-rounded support that extends far beyond dialysis sessions.

Strengthening Communication Channels

One of the most important ways case managers foster collaboration is by establishing clear communication channels. Regular team meetings, daily huddles, and care conferences allow healthcare professionals to share updates, discuss complications, and align treatment strategies. For example, if a patient develops high blood pressure despite dietary adjustments, the dietitian, nephrologist, and pharmacist can collaboratively identify causes and solutions, coordinated by the case manager. This open exchange of information prevents missteps, builds trust, and enhances the quality of care delivery.

Dialysis Champions

Facilitating Care Transitions

Dialysis patients often move between hospital stays, outpatient dialysis centers, and home care. These transitions are fraught with risks, such as medication errors or missed follow-up appointments. Case managers take ownership of this process by coordinating discharge planning, reconciling medication lists, and arranging home health services when necessary. They also ensure that follow-up appointments are scheduled and communicated clearly. By managing these transitions, case managers prevent gaps in care, reduce readmission rates, and support smoother recoveries.

Engaging Patients and Caregivers

Collaboration is incomplete without including the patient and their caregivers. Case managers actively involve them in care planning, goal setting, and decision-making. This engagement not only strengthens adherence to treatment but also promotes shared decision-making. For example, when a patient struggles with fluid restrictions, the case manager may involve family members in learning meal preparation techniques, reinforcing the patient's ability to stick to dietary guidelines. By empowering patients and caregivers to take ownership of their health, case managers cultivate a sense of partnership that enhances long-term outcomes.

Uncovering the Root Causes of Dialysis Needs

Transforming Healthcare Through Case Management

When patient advocacy and interdisciplinary collaboration intersect, the result is transformative. Case managers create an environment where patients feel respected, healthcare professionals work in unison, and care is delivered with safety and compassion at its core.

Advocating for patient rights ensures that healthcare is not only about treating illness but also about respecting dignity, autonomy, and choice. At the same time, fostering collaboration ensures that the system works as one cohesive unit, delivering care that is coordinated, consistent, and comprehensive. Together, these roles elevate dialysis care from a technical procedure to a holistic healthcare journey.

In the broader context of healthcare reform, case managers represent a model for the future: professionals who connect systems, empower patients, and improve outcomes through advocacy and collaboration. By embedding these practices into daily dialysis care, healthcare systems can move closer to their ultimate goal—delivering care that is safe, equitable, patient-centered, and transformative.

Medication Reconciliation: Building a Safe Foundation

The cornerstone of medication safety in dialysis care is thorough medication reconciliation. Patients with kidney disease often see multiple specialists, and their medication lists can be long, complicated, and constantly changing. This makes them especially vulnerable to discrepancies and errors.

Case managers conduct comprehensive reviews of each patient's medications, carefully examining the list of drugs, dosages, frequency, route of administration, and patterns of adherence. They identify duplications, outdated prescriptions, or dangerous drug-drug interactions that may otherwise go unnoticed. For example, certain blood pressure medications may interact with drugs used to treat anemia, leading to unanticipated side effects if not carefully monitored.

By systematically checking for contraindications and potential adverse effects, case managers reduce the risk of medical errors and provide a solid foundation for safe and effective treatment. This meticulous approach not only protects patients from harm but also gives healthcare teams confidence that prescribed regimens are accurate and aligned with patients' clinical needs.

Uncovering the Root Causes of Dialysis Needs

Medication Education: Empowering Patients with Knowledge

Once a safe regimen has been established, case managers turn their attention to patient education. Many patients undergoing dialysis are prescribed more than a dozen medications, each with its own indications, actions, precautions, and side effects. Without proper understanding, patients may misuse medications, skip doses, or abandon treatment altogether.

Case managers provide clear, accessible explanations of each prescribed medication. They discuss why the drug is necessary, how it works, potential side effects, and strategies for recognizing and managing complications. Patients are also educated on practical aspects such as administration techniques, safe storage requirements, and the importance of consistency in timing and dosage.

For instance, a patient may need to take phosphate binders with meals to prevent mineral imbalances, but if they do not understand this requirement, the drug's effectiveness diminishes. By clarifying such details, case managers empower patients to take control of their own care.

Education also extends to family members and caregivers. By involving them in discussions, case managers ensure that the patient's support network is equipped to reinforce safe medication practices at home. In this way, education becomes both an empowering tool and a preventive measure against errors.

Medication Coordination: Ensuring Access and Continuity

Even the most well-designed medication regimen is useless if patients cannot consistently access their prescriptions. Barriers such as insurance restrictions, prior authorization requirements, or specialty pharmacy delays can disrupt continuity of care and compromise health outcomes.

Case managers act as coordinators, collaborating closely with healthcare providers, pharmacists, and other care team members to streamline medication processes. They ensure timely refills, renewals, and authorizations are in place so patients never miss critical doses. In cases where specialty pharmacy services are needed—for example, for injectable medications—case managers arrange delivery, train patients on safe administration, and confirm that necessary supplies are available.

Additionally, case managers serve as problem-solvers when unexpected issues arise. If a medication is suddenly out of stock, too expensive, or no longer covered by insurance, they work with providers to identify safe alternatives. Their proactive coordination minimizes disruptions, ensures continuity, and reduces the risk of complications or hospitalizations related to medication gaps.

Medication Adherence: Overcoming Barriers and Building Habits

One of the most significant challenges in dialysis care is medication adherence. Patients often struggle with complex regimens, financial burdens, cultural beliefs, or side effects that make adherence difficult. Left unaddressed, nonadherence can lead to disease progression, complications, and costly hospitalizations.

Case managers play a central role in identifying and addressing these barriers. They conduct assessments to determine why patients may struggle with adherence—whether it is forgetfulness, literacy limitations, financial strain, or skepticism about the treatment's effectiveness. With this insight, they develop tailored strategies to support each individual.

For example, patients who forget doses may benefit from pill organizers, reminder phone calls, or digital applications that send alerts. Those struggling with costs may be connected to patient assistance programs or insurance navigation support. If side effects deter patients from continuing their regimen, case managers collaborate with healthcare providers to adjust dosages or switch medications.

Cultural beliefs and health literacy are also important considerations. Some patients may hesitate to take medications due to cultural norms, spiritual practices, or mistrust of healthcare systems. Case managers use cultural sensitivity and plain-language explanations to address these concerns respectfully, ensuring that patients feel understood and supported rather than judged.

By implementing such strategies, case managers transform medication adherence from a daily struggle into a manageable routine. Over time, this leads to better health outcomes, reduced hospitalizations, and a stronger sense of patient empowerment.

Case Managers as Agents of Transformation in Healthcare

The role of case managers in dialysis medication management goes beyond simply checking prescriptions. They act as educators, coordinators, advocates, and problem-solvers—ensuring that every aspect of a patient's medication regimen is safe, accessible, and sustainable. Their work has profound implications for transforming healthcare in several ways:

1. **Improved Safety:** By conducting thorough medication reconciliations, case managers reduce the risk of harmful

interactions, duplications, or omissions.

2. **Patient Empowerment:** Through education, patients gain the knowledge and confidence to manage their medications responsibly.

3. **Continuity of Care:** By coordinating refills, renewals, and specialty services, case managers prevent dangerous interruptions in treatment.

4. **Reduced Costs:** By improving adherence and preventing complications, case managers help lower the rates of hospitalizations and emergency interventions.

5. **Holistic Support:** By addressing cultural, financial, and personal barriers, case managers treat patients as whole individuals, not just clinical cases.

Performance Monitoring: Tracking Progress for Better Outcomes

One of the most essential responsibilities of case managers is **performance monitoring**. They continuously assess key performance indicators (KPIs) and clinical outcomes to ensure that dialysis patients receive the highest standard of care. These indicators include:

- Dialysis adequacy

- Vascular access management
- Infection rates
- Hospitalization rates
- Mortality rates
- Patient satisfaction scores

By using tools such as data analytics platforms, electronic health records (EHRs), and quality reporting systems, case managers can detect trends, highlight performance gaps, and measure progress over time. For example, a rising infection rate may signal gaps in infection control practices, while declining patient satisfaction scores may reveal communication or care delivery issues. Proactive monitoring allows case managers to identify problems early and address them before they escalate, ultimately improving patient safety and well-being.

Root Cause Analysis: Preventing Problems Before They Recur

When problems occur, case managers lead or participate in **root cause analysis (RCA)** to uncover the underlying factors contributing to adverse events or poor outcomes. Rather than simply treating symptoms of a problem, RCA seeks to identify its true source.

Uncovering the Root Causes of Dialysis Needs

Techniques often used include:

- **Fishbone diagrams:** Mapping out possible causes of a problem such as treatment delays or medication errors.
- **Process mapping:** Visualizing workflows to identify inefficiencies or breakdowns in communication.
- **Failure Mode and Effects Analysis (FMEA):** Predicting potential points of failure in dialysis care and ranking them by severity and likelihood.

For example, if treatment non-adherence is common among patients, RCA may reveal underlying causes such as poor health literacy, transportation challenges, or side effects. Once these causes are identified, targeted interventions—such as transportation services, medication education, or alternative treatment options—can be implemented to reduce recurrence.

Continuous Quality Improvement: Embedding Excellence in Care

Beyond identifying and solving immediate issues, case managers promote a culture of **continuous quality improvement (CQI)**. This involves developing, implementing, and evaluating long-term initiatives that enhance both clinical outcomes and patient experience.

Case managers often:

- Participate in **task forces and interdisciplinary teams** to standardize best practices.
- Lead **audits and performance reviews** to evaluate current processes.
- Implement evidence-based practices to improve care protocols.
- Foster collaboration with all stakeholders to ensure broad engagement.

For example, introducing standardized protocols for vascular access care can reduce complications across the patient population, while patient education programs can improve treatment adherence.

Patient Feedback: The Heart of Quality Care

To ensure dialysis care is not only clinically effective but also patient-centered, case managers integrate **patient feedback** into quality improvement efforts. Feedback is gathered through surveys, focus groups, and direct discussions with patients, caregivers, and families.

By listening to patient experiences, case managers can identify gaps in service delivery, such as:

- Long waiting times

- Communication barriers
- Lack of psychosocial support
- Insufficient education about treatment options

Integrating this feedback fosters transparency, accountability, and responsiveness within the healthcare system. Moreover, it ensures that patients' voices shape the quality initiatives that directly affect their care.

Algorithm Overview

Case managers follow a structured, step-by-step approach to ensure holistic, effective, and patient-centered dialysis care. This algorithm provides a roadmap for their work.

Step 1: Assessing Patient Needs

Initial Assessment:

Case managers begin with a thorough review of the patient's medical history, current health status, and psychosocial factors. This step helps identify both clinical and non-clinical needs.

Ongoing Evaluation:

Regular check-ins allow case managers to track changes in health status, treatment response, or personal circumstances, ensuring care plans remain relevant and effective.

Step 2: Developing Personalized Care Plans

Interdisciplinary Collaboration:

Case managers work closely with nephrologists, nurses, dietitians, and social workers to design individualized care plans.

Holistic Approach:

These plans go beyond clinical treatment by addressing nutrition, mental health, and social services, ensuring patients receive comprehensive support.

Step 3: Coordinating with Healthcare Providers

Seamless Care Transitions:

Case managers play a vital role in moving patients safely between care settings, such as hospital discharges or shifts to home dialysis.

Streamlined Communication:

By keeping providers aligned and informed, case managers reduce duplication of efforts, miscommunication, and treatment delays.

Step 4: Monitoring Patient Progress

Tracking Health Indicators:

Case managers closely monitor blood pressure, hemoglobin levels, and dialysis adequacy to ensure treatments are effective.

Uncovering the Root Causes of Dialysis Needs

Treatment Adherence:

Non-adherence is a common challenge in dialysis care. Case managers identify barriers—such as cost, fatigue, or side effects—and provide strategies to overcome them.

Outcome Evaluation:

Regular evaluations ensure the care plan is achieving its intended results and allow adjustments when needed.

Step 5: Educating Patients and Caregivers

Comprehensive Education:

Patients and caregivers are taught about treatment options, medication safety, and the importance of adherence.

Lifestyle Modifications:

Case managers provide guidance on diet, exercise, and stress management, which are essential for improving long-term outcomes.

Patient Engagement:

By encouraging patients to actively participate in their care, case managers foster self-efficacy and greater treatment success.

Step 6: Advocating for Patients' Rights

Equitable Access:

Case managers ensure all patients have equal access to necessary care and support services, regardless of socioeconomic status or background.

Patient Preferences:

Respect for autonomy is central. Patients' values and preferences are incorporated into care planning and decision-making.

Liaison Role:

Case managers act as intermediaries between patients and healthcare organizations, ensuring patient concerns are heard and addressed.

www.ingramcontent.com/pod-product-compliance
Lightning Source LLC
Chambersburg PA
CBHW052027030426
42337CB00027B/4890